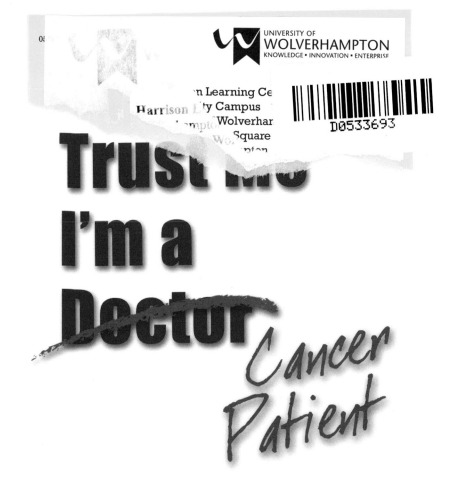

Trust Me I'm a Doctor *Cancer Patient*

Dr Wesley C Finegan

MB BCh BAO MRCGP MICGP D Pall Med

Radcliffe Medical Press

Oxford • San Francisco

Radcliffe Medical Press Ltd
18 Marcham Road
Abingdon
Oxon OX14 1AA
United Kingdom

www.radcliffe-oxford.com
The Radcliffe Medical Press electronic catalogue and online ordering facility.
Direct sales to anywhere in the world.

British Library Cataloguing in Publication Data

A catalogue record for this book is available from the British Library.

ISBN 1 85775 877 3

Typeset by Anne Joshua & Associates, Oxford
Printed and bound by TJ International Ltd, Padstow, Cornwall

Contents

About the author

I was aged three when I first announced that I wanted to be a doctor. In 1978 I achieved that aim when I qualified from The Queen's University of Belfast. After a further four years of training, I entered general practice in East Sussex.

Over the next nine years I developed an increasing interest in caring for patients with cancer and this led to my being appointed as a consultant in palliative medicine in central Scotland in 1991.

In 1994 I became a cancer patient myself and had to retire from my hospice post on the grounds of ill health. I was very fortunate to be offered a post with the University of Dundee where I continue to offer some input into their courses on cancer and palliative care.

In 1979 Alice and I were married and we have two children, Chris and Sharon.

Wesley C Finegan
August 2003

Acknowledgements

I acknowledge, with gratitude, the help and advice offered by Patricia Manson BDS with the chapters 'I have a dry mouth' and 'I have a sore mouth'.

I thank Mr Christopher Reeve for his kind permission to use the quotation in the Introduction on page vii.

My thanks also to the doctors and nurses who allowed me to work in tandem with them, to all the people who offered constructive feedback, to my family for their patience during the writing and to the many patients who taught me so much over the years.

Introduction

When I was diagnosed with cancer in 1994, someone said to me, 'You will cope better because you know what to expect.'

Actually, I did not know what to expect. I had never been a cancer patient before.

This book is primarily written for cancer sufferers, although patients with other illnesses may suffer the same problems and might find some of the ideas here of value.

Knowing a bit about cancer helped me to work with the doctors and nurses and set realistic, achievable goals.

Let me quote from the *British Medical Journal* earlier this year:[1]

Christopher Reeve never used to visit a doctor; now he relies on doctors and carers continually for his survival and wellbeing. So what makes a good doctor? And a good patient?

Mr Reeve said, 'I think that today we are in a new era of medicine, one that is very different from the old. The old way, it used to be that the doctors were the experts, and the patients knew nothing and were expected to rely on the doctors' expertise – literally, "the doctor knows best".

'It's giving the patient control and developing a partnership with the patient. That is clearly the way to go. Doctors and patients really need to collaborate on reversing illness and disability or achieving the best possible outcome.'

Hopefully this book will help you to collaborate and achieve the best outcome for a variety of distressing symptoms.

Reference

1 Eaton L (2003) Man and Superman – patients in control: the way to go. *BMJ*. **326**: 1287–90. (Reproduced with the kind permission of Mr Christopher Reeve and Lynn Eaton.)

How do you use this book?

Before you start, let me say two things. First, just because something is included in this book it does not imply that you will necessarily experience the problem.

Secondly, issues will be raised that you have not thought about. Some of these could be threatening to read, so don't try to handle these problems until you are ready.

This is a practical book – to be consulted frequently, not read and put on the shelf. To use the book effectively, you also need a notebook and a pen. Each problem or symptom discussed is dealt with under six headings and you are invited to think and make your own notes. Hopefully these will help you when you are discussing that problem with the nurse or doctor.

When I was a small boy, I saw a strange thing. It was a bicycle with two riders. One was steering, but both were pedalling! I asked my mother what it was. She explained that it was a tandem – a bicycle built for two.

When we think about our journey along the cancer road, the concept of the tandem fits well. By sharing the experiences of others and myself, hopefully we can work 'in tandem' and I can steer you along the unknown route ahead. I remind you that both parties have to do some pedalling!

The content is the product of my diaries, discussions, personal experience and the shared experiences of other patients. It is intended to help you on your personal cancer journey and to encourage you to work with the doctors, nurses and others who will be caring for you. I hope you find it useful.

How can we work 'in TANDEM'?

Each chapter in this book is broken down into the following sections.

The doctor says

Here I will give you some relevant information to help you understand more about the symptom being discussed.

We then use the word TANDEM to examine the various issues from different aspects.

T Think

Often, when asked a question, I had to stop and think before I answered. Hopefully by thinking beforehand, you can prepare for the kinds of questions a nurse or doctor might ask you.

A Ask

When I got home, I often thought of something I had meant to ask. Here you will find some issues you might wish to raise when you are invited to ask questions.

N Note

Making a note of a relevant detail now might save you a lot of difficulty remembering in a few weeks' time!

D Do

Here you'll find practical ideas that have been tried and tested by my patients and by me.

E Explore

Sometimes we want to know more or find out about something we would like to know about. I'll try and guide you to the best sources of information. If I am aware of a good resource, I'll include it, but I do not claim to know them all!

M More Information

If there is something that has not been said already and it's relevant, you'll find it here.

For Alice, who learned of her own cancer
just before this book went to press.

Pain

Chapter 1

How can my pain be assessed?

The doctor says

Before we look at the very complex subject of pain, bear with me as I explain a few things that might help you understand what the doctor and nurse are trying to do.

What exactly is 'pain'?

This may sound a pretty daft question, but it is actually one that nurses and doctors spend lots of time thinking about. We will also look at some questions you might feel like asking.

Pain is a very complex problem. You will be well aware that there are many different kinds of pain. For example, toothache is very different from the aches and pains you associate with an afternoon moving heavy furniture or digging the garden.

There are many definitions of 'pain' in medical textbooks. Some go into great detail about what exactly is going on inside to cause the pain: others try and describe the pain in words. At the end of the day, the definition I like best is: 'Pain is whatever the patient says hurts.'

Lots of things may be 'hurting you' just now. You may be in pain in a part of your body – so that hurts in the form of *physical* pain. You may have no physical pain whatsoever, but be hurting *emotionally* because of your illness and what it is doing to you. It's almost certain that your illness is having an impact on family life and relationships with friends, so you are hurting *socially*. Whether you are religious or not, you might be wondering why this is happening, what it all means and possibly wondering why God is allowing it to happen – that's *spiritual* pain. Therefore, taken as a whole, you may be hurting in any of four ways. These four make up your 'total hurting' or 'total pain'.

We will look at emotional, social and spiritual pain in the chapter 'I am "hurting" because of my illness' (*see* Chapter 33). The aim of this chapter is to help you describe your physical pain and to tell you something about how the doctor or nurse assesses your pain and decides the best way to deal with it.

Why try and measure the amount of pain I have?

You have a very important part to play in the management of your pain. Only you know how severe your pain is and what it is like.

You might have more than one pain. That's something you might not want to mention – you might think it sounds strange. I have had several patients who have had three different pains at the same time. If my patients had only talked about one of these, the other two might not have been dealt with. Mention all the pains you have – if you don't you might not get the most suitable treatment.

How can the amount of pain you have be measured or assessed?

You will be asked several questions, or you might possibly be asked to fill in a sheet of questions. Don't worry: there are no 'wrong answers'. What you feel and how you feel it is unique to you. Don't be afraid to say what *you* are feeling.

The questions you will be asked are designed to find out the following kinds of information:

- What makes your pain start and what helps it get better?
- What is your pain like?
- Where is your pain and does it go anywhere else?
- How bad is your pain?
- When do you get your pain?

Let's think about these, taking a typical question from each category.

Think

Typical question: What makes your pain start, or get worse?

Lots of things may make your pain come on. Think of what makes your pain start or get worse and tick all the boxes that apply.

☐	Anxiety or worry
☐	Exercise
☐	Movement
☐	Sitting too long
☐	Standing
☐	Tiredness
☐	No obvious reason
☐	Other (write it down here)

Typical question: What makes your pain get better?

☐	Feeling relaxed and confident
☐	Lying down
☐	Moving around
☐	Rest or sleep
☐	Sitting down
☐	Tablets/medicine
☐	Other (write it down here)

Typical question: What is your pain like?

Don't forget to describe each pain.

Your description of your pain is very important. Since the doctor or nurse can't feel your pain, they depend on your description of it. This is not always easy, so here are some words that have been used to describe pain. One book I have lists hundreds of other words that have been used. Don't worry: there are no 'right' or 'wrong' words, just try and describe your pain by ticking the word or words that best describe your pain(s).

If you have more than one pain, make a note of where this pain is beside its description.

☐	Aching
☐	Burning
☐	Crushing
☐	Deep
☐	Dull
☐	Like electric shocks
☐	Gnawing
☐	Heavy
☐	Like a knife
☐	Stabbing
☐	Tight
☐	Tingling
☐	Vice-like
☐	Other (describe)

You might be thinking, 'The more pains I describe, the more tablets I'll be given.' That's logical, but thankfully it's not always like that. It is important to describe all your pains because it helps determine the exact cause and that makes it easier to choose the best medication to suit all your pains.

Typical question: Where is your pain and does it go anywhere else?

To help you, here are two body diagrams. Use a different coloured pen for each of your pains to mark where they are and if they go anywhere else.

When you look at these pictures, you might think they are the wrong way round, but they're not! It's just the same as when you are looking at someone standing in front of you. I have marked the right and left sides of the body to help you.

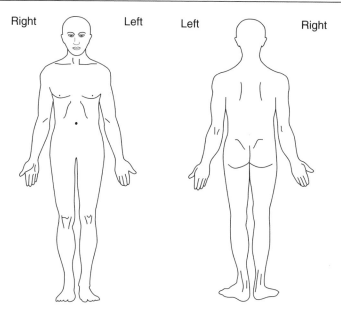

Fig. 1.1 Body diagrams for marking sites of pain.

(These diagrams are reproduced at the end of the book for you to copy)

Typical question: How bad is your pain?

This can be difficult to answer. Doctors and nurses sometimes use a variety of ways to try and measure pain. These are called 'pain assessment tools'. Some of these are questionnaires, and some are measuring scales like small rulers that you mark to show how bad your pain is. There are several of these and I will describe a couple of the common ones in the section 'More Information'.

It is probably easiest at this stage for you to describe your pain in your own words like 'no pain', 'mild pain', 'moderate pain' or 'severe pain'. Do not try to decide how much pain is 'mild' or 'severe'. What matters is, how do *you* feel about *your* pain? The amount of pain you feel is unique to you and nobody can say that you have too much or too little pain.

Typical question: When do you get your pain?

This is really about whether your pain is constant or whether it comes and goes. If it comes and goes, think about when it comes on and when it eases. Does a particular action or movement bring it on; is it worse or better at night? Does it seem to start at a particular time of day for no apparent reason? These questions need to be answered for all the pains you have.

If you are not in pain at the moment, it might be better for you to complete this section the next time you have pain.

Ask

- Look at the lists under the 'Think' section. If you are suffering pain, your present medication may need to be reviewed. Ask about this.
- Ask how soon to expect relief of your pain after your medication has been reviewed.
- Is your pain made worse, or brought on, by activities that are essential but are becoming difficult for you? You might wish to ask your GP if there is help available.

Note

You have already made most of your notes by ticking the boxes in the 'Think' section, but you should make a note of the effectiveness of any changes to your current medication and whether there are any side effects. If you do experience side effects, report them.

Do

- Try and avoid unnecessary activities that make your pain worse.
- Accept help if it is offered.
- Take your medication exactly as prescribed and tell the nurse or doctor if it is not giving you the relief you expected after the time when it was thought it should be effective.

Explore

I am not going to recommend that you start trying to become an expert on the drugs that are used to relieve pain. You would need many years of hard study to achieve that goal!

It follows, therefore, that I do not recommend you explore all kinds of unfounded claims seen on TV or the Internet. Don't waste time and money and put yourself at risk trying some untested drug that might interfere with what you are taking already!

If you choose to explore the value of acupuncture or acupressure or any other complementary therapy (*see* Chapter 38), by all means do so, but do not start any course of treatment without consulting your doctor first. Be aware that some of these treatments may not be available free on the NHS, can be quite expensive and may involve travelling.

More Information 📖

There are several kinds of 'pain assessment tool' used to measure pain. The common ones are:

- **A number scale**: You choose a number between 0 and 10 to describe how bad your pain is.

0

No pain

                                             10

Worst pain

If you are not in pain, this scores a zero and the worst pain you can imagine scores 10. Patients sometimes say, 'I don't know what is the worst pain imaginable.' That's OK – it's how you think your pain is. If you can't imagine the pain being any worse, say so. Nobody is asking you to be an expert on how bad pain can be. Just put down what you think, but don't be afraid to ask for advice.

- **A linear scale**: This is a straight line, usually 10 cm long, marked 'no pain' at one end and something like 'worst pain possible' at the other. You mark the line where you think your pain is on this line.

No pain   **Worst pain**

The purpose of these scales is not to see how good you are at judging pain but to record, on a series of charts, whether your pain is getting better or worse. Because you are the person who is judging the severity of the pain, *you* know what you mean and you are the best person to tell the nurse and doctor how your pain is doing.

The value of using any of these tools is to check regularly that the amount of pain you have is decreasing, with the aim of getting you free of pain as soon as possible.

We all feel pain differently. This is just a fact of life and you are not 'weak' just because you feel pain. Equally importantly, do not try to appear 'strong' by refusing to admit to how much pain you feel.

A couple of other thoughts about pain

You are unique and how you feel pain is unique to you. Pain can vary during the day for no apparent reason. I have found that I could have a good day with almost no pain and then have another day when, for no apparent reason, I was much less comfortable. This can't always be explained, but as I said earlier there are some things that make your pain feel worse. These include boredom, depression (*see* Chapter 11), discomfort, fear, loneliness, sadness (*see* Chapter 40), sleeplessness (*see* Chapter 22) and worry. If you can identify some of these as relating to you, ask about them. They might be affecting how much pain you are feeling.

Chapter 2

What do I need to know about my pain?

The doctor says

You are probably thinking, 'I don't want to know about my pain, just let them treat it!' Even so, there are a few issues that are worth thinking about.

Think

How much do you want to know about your pain? Are you interested in what is causing it or how it will be treated? You probably don't want too much detail, so that's good, for I am not writing a textbook! There are a few things worth considering.

- How many pains have you got? Have you mentioned them all?
- Think about whether you want to ask about your pain. If you do, please read on.

Ask

If you have more than one type of pain, you will need to ask the same questions for each type of pain.

Tick any boxes that apply so that you can quickly check what you need to ask about.

☐	What is causing your pain? You might already know this, but your pain might not be directly caused by the cancer. Other painful problems like arthritis don't go away when cancer is diagnosed.
☐	How long will it be before the treatment starts to work?
☐	What do you do if the pain has not improved within this time frame?
☐	You might wish to ask about your ability to drive when taking strong painkillers. Some painkillers can make you sleepy for a day or two. Ask for advice about driving and whether you need to tell the DVLA or your insurance company that you are taking this medication. (The 'small print' often states that you are not insured when you are on medication that could affect your ability to drive.) *See* 'More Information' for some more detail about this.

Note

It can be difficult to remember which treatments worked and which caused side effects. You might find it helpful to keep a note of how bad your pain was before you started any treatment and how much better it was with the treatment you were given. Keep a note of any side effects too.

Keep the original containers or copy the details from the bottle or box of painkillers and make a note of their effectiveness and any side effects you experienced.

Do

The main thing to do is to try and keep accurate records of how your pain responds to each treatment and not to be afraid to admit that a particular treatment did not help. This is sometimes called a 'pain diary'. To keep your own pain diary, use the following type of format.

☐ Day and date
☐ Where was the pain?
☐ How bad was the pain (describe all your pains)?
☐ What seemed to make it come on/get worse?
☐ What was it like?
☐ When did it start?
☐ How long did it last?
☐ Any extra medication taken?
☐ How well did it respond to the medication?
☐ What else did you do to ease the pain?

The doctor or nurse will find this information useful in assessing your pain and the medicines used to treat it. There are many different types of painkiller and sometimes it takes time to find the one that suits you best.

If you don't accurately report what happens to you, you could end up suffering for no reason. Nobody will be angry when you tell them that something didn't work – it is all part of the process of effective pain assessment and management.

On the other hand, there are some people who want to have some pain so that they can 'monitor their disease progress'. If this is what you wish to do, say so. It is your right to decide what you want, but do tell the nurses and doctors what you are doing so that you both work together to achieve the same goal. If you don't say what you are doing, it could be interpreted as not complying with instructions!

At the back of this book is a sheet that you can copy and use as the basis of your pain diary.

Explore

There is not a lot to explore by yourself. I am aware of all kinds of cures and treatments being advertised. Many of these are misleading and some are blatantly untrue. Some medicines advertised have not been fully tested. They may contain extra ingredients that are not listed and some of these can react with the medications you have been prescribed. It's simply not worth the risk, or the cost, when anything you need will almost always be provided free on the NHS.

TENS machines are frequently advertised. They suit some types of pain very well, but have no effect on other pains. Ask for advice, from someone treating you, before spending your money. Asking the advertiser will almost certainly result in your buying the product!

If you do choose to try something, please do not do so without telling the doctor. You should also be aware that detailed information on many products bought from herbalists, health stores, over the Internet or from newspaper or television advertisements is simply not made readily available to the medical profession. The doctor will not always be able to confirm that a bought product is safe to take in combination with a prescribed medicine.

More Information 📖

Accurate assessment of your pain is an important part of managing your pain. It's easy to think that one painkiller will relieve all pains. This is not always the case, especially for cancer pain. Most pains can be relieved: the secret is in finding out about the pain first – what it's like, what is causing it and how bad it is. With this information, which can only be provided by you, the most suitable medicine is chosen and the dose is carefully calculated for your individual needs.

It is not uncommon for more than one type of painkiller to be required to control pain. This is not something to worry about and does not suggest that things are out of control.

What about driving when taking strong painkillers?

The DVLA

The situation with the DVLA is as follows (January 2003):

- **For a normal (class 1) driving licence**: Notification of cancer is required ONLY if:
  - you develop problems with your nervous system
  - treatment or weakness prevents normal daily activities
  - medication causes side effects likely to affect safe driving.
- **For a LGV (class 2) driving licence**: Notification of cancer is required if the following types of cancer have been diagnosed in the past two years:
  - lung
  - melanoma
  - lymphoma.

In addition, one must advise the DVLA of 'any other medical condition likely to affect ability to safely control a vehicle, e.g. amputation, impairment secondary to medication, chronic debilitation or illness'.

The DVLA web site www.dvla.gov.uk/drivers/dmed1 offers updated information about notifiable medical conditions.

Insurance

Since it is possible that strong painkillers could cause impaired or delayed reactions or drowsiness, my advice would be that you should report your condition and advise of any strong painkiller currently being prescribed before you continue to drive. Your insurance company may have their own guidance and it is impossible to give an accurate statement here that covers all the companies' individual policies.

Chapter 3

What do I need to know about the treatment for my pain?

The doctor says

There are many different medications used for pain. Explaining how and why they work would require several very large textbooks! Trust me while I give one or two simple examples and trust the doctor when you are offered something that is not usually prescribed for pain.

Pain is generated when nerve endings are stimulated by direct damage or pressure, or by a change in the surrounding tissues. Nerves are hollow pipes filled with a fluid that conducts electricity. Chemical changes in the fluid inside the nerve or in the tissues around the nerve generate minute amounts of electricity. This electricity is carried along the nerve to the brain. There are several types of nerve and, depending on the type of nerve stimulated, the electrical current will be interpreted as heat, cold, sharp pain, dull ache, burning sensations, or even itch.

The basic way in which painkillers act is either to neutralise the chemical changes in the tissue or to stop the electrical signal from reaching the brain.

Most of us have taken ibuprofen at some time for pain or after an injury. It works by neutralising a chemical produced in injured tissues. When the chemical is neutralised, the electrical signals are no longer produced and the pain eases.

Most of us will know of someone who suffers from epileptic fits. Fits are caused by an abnormal electrical signal being generated in the brain. The tablets used for fits can also stop electrical impulses travelling along nerves going to the brain and thus can stop us feeling certain types of pain.

Choosing the right drug is a matter of experience on the part of the doctor and also your accurate reporting of your pain.

To complicate matters even more, there are also nerves that inhibit the transfer of pain impulses to the brain! TENS machines work by activating these inhibitory nerves, but TENS only works for certain types of pain.

So, pain is a pretty complex subject!

Think

- How many different pains can you identify that affect you at present? Some of these might respond to the same painkiller, but, if not, you might need more than one medication.
- Have you been taking painkillers that have helped one pain but not another? If so, tell the doctor or nurse about this.

- Have the painkillers been helping your pain but causing unpleasant side effects? If so, report this to the doctor. A minor change in your medicines will probably relieve the pain without causing other problems.

Ask

You will obviously be told the name of the medication you are given. Sometimes there is an information leaflet included with the tablets or medicine. Read this, but think about any other things that you might need to know. Here are a few thoughts.

- You might want to ask whether your medicine has any significant side effects and what these are.
- Can you continue driving while taking this medication?
- How long before the drug should be effective?
- What do you do if the medication is not working within this time?

Note

Make a note of any medication that you are given, what it was for, how well it worked and any problems you had with it. Keep a note of when you started taking any new medicines and when any new problems began. This becomes even more important when you are taking several different tablets, because it helps identify when a problem arises and whether it is in any way associated with a new medication.

Do

It's time to state the obvious!

- Take your medication exactly as you are told to do.
- Do not listen to alternative advice from anyone who is not involved in your healthcare.
- Don't take anything else without asking the doctor, nurse or pharmacist first.

It makes sense to always try and get your medications from the same pharmacist. They keep a list of the medicines you are taking and can offer you excellent advice. They can only do this if they know about your prescription, so be fair and don't go to a different shop and ask the pharmacist there for advice.

Before buying other medications over the counter, ask for advice from the pharmacist who dispenses your prescriptions. Some items that can be bought over the counter should not be taken with the medications you have been prescribed.

Explore

Ask your pharmacist about tablet boxes with multiple compartments that allow you to organise your tablets to be taken at various times throughout the day. Some can be filled for seven days at a time.

You will find lots of information about any medication you are prescribed, especially if you search the Internet. Who wrote it?

If you want to explore more about medicines used to control pain, I suggest that you only consult books written by suitably qualified professionals or look at web sites such as www.cancerbacup.org.uk which is the CancerBACUP web site.

More Information

Managing pain is a complex task, best undertaken by trained professionals. Your doctor will be well equipped to manage most of the pain problems that present, but for the more difficult problems there are pain specialists, often working in pain clinics in hospital. Research into pain and how to manage it is a rapidly advancing area.

Don't panic if you are offered an appointment at a pain clinic – it is one way to ensure that you are offered the best advice from someone who is up-to-date with new research and experienced in dealing with the kind of problem you have.

Chapter 4

What else do I need to know about pain management?

The doctor says

As a doctor with a special interest in managing pain, I can tell you that you don't need to know much about the science of pain management, but you do need to obey the instructions you are given! Having said that you don't need to know much, here are a few things that are useful to know.

There are six basic principles that doctors and nurses try to adopt in managing pain.

1 How treatment is given

Treatment is usually given in tablet or liquid form. We try to avoid injections, but this is not always possible and occasionally a 'syringe driver' may be used to deliver tiny regular amounts of painkilling drugs by injection.

Sometimes patches may be applied to the skin, or sometimes suppositories are inserted into the rectum (back passage) to avoid upsetting a delicate stomach.

See Chapter 5 'Some questions frequently asked about pain' for more details about syringe drivers and the use of skin patches for pain.

2 When treatment is given

Painkillers are usually given regularly because pain tends to recur as soon as the effect of the tablets wears off. The usual advice is for you to take your medication at regular intervals so that pain is kept under control as much as possible.

3 The medication dose is adjusted as required to keep your pain under control

Sometimes it can be anticipated that pain might get worse. In these cases, you might be given something to take when you need it if your pain becomes worse. This is called a 'breakthrough dose'. If you need frequent breakthrough doses, let the nurse or doctor know how much extra you need on an average day. Your regular doses might need to be adjusted slightly so that you can be pain free.

Similarly, as pain improves, the doses will be reduced.

In practical terms, these situations can result in your having several boxes or bottles of the same tablets, but all of different strengths. Make sure you know which one you are currently taking. It's very easy to make a mistake.

4 Medication is prescribed according to your individual needs

The medication you were given is for you – not someone else. Don't share or swap! It's tempting to compare your medicines with those of another patient, but it's not going to help and might only confuse you! Trust the doctor or nurse!

5 A second drug might be used – if appropriate

It is a popular belief that one painkiller should kill all pains. Sadly this belief is untrue and sometimes a second drug is needed. These might not be painkillers in their own right but act with the painkillers to relieve the pain more effectively.

6 **Everything is prescribed with attention to detail**

It's easy to become worried about the number of tablets or the strength of the tablets you are being given. Do not worry. Everything is carefully calculated and checked and nobody wants you to be taking any medication for longer than you need it.

Think

If you have been exploring and finding out about pain, you might be aware that there are treatments advertised that do not appear to be available locally. It is impossible to offer every service in every local hospital, so for some treatments you might have to travel to a bigger hospital some distance away. Now you have to think a little.

- How do you feel about trying different treatments – is it worth the travelling? In most cases, you will be offered what is most suitable for you, but you might be willing to travel to a bigger hospital or specialist centre for specialised treatments. Travelling is tiring, especially if the treatment requires frequent attendance.
- What are your feelings about complementary (alternative) medicine? Homoe-opathy, acupuncture and a variety of other complementary therapies are available on the NHS, but there may not be suitably qualified practitioners working for the NHS in your area. You might have to pay, or be prepared to travel quite a distance to be offered these services.

Ask

It is worth asking about the treatments you are being offered for your pain.

- How soon will it work?
- What do you do if you are still in pain after this time, or there has been no effect at all?
- What are the likely side effects (if any)?
- If you might experience side effects, are they likely to be very troublesome, and what can be done about this?
- Is it worth the time, effort and expense of trying complementary therapies such as acupuncture?

Note

Make a note of how well the medication helps your pain. The aim is to get you free of pain and keep you free of pain most of the time, if not all of the time. In practice, there might be some activities that cause you some pain for a short time, e.g. exercise. You may be able to cope with this without extra painkillers. Keep a 'pain diary' as described in Chapter 2 'What do I need to know about my pain?' This information will be of great value to the doctor or nurse.

Do

At the risk of repeating myself, take your medication *exactly* as you were told to. That is the most important thing to do.

You should also set realistic targets for yourself, noting what brings on your pain. If you can avoid these activities, do so. If you can't avoid them, try and break them into smaller or shorter activities that are less demanding, with a short rest between each exercise, and see if that allows you to remain active but pain free. If this does not work, make a note and discuss this with the doctor.

Explore

You might wish to explore the availability of complementary therapies in your area. Do so by all means, but do not start any course of treatment and do not take any form of medication, even herbal, unless you have first discussed it with the doctor who is looking after you.

Be aware of clever advertising that offers a variety of appliances that might make life easier for you. They are almost always expensive and you won't know how helpful they are until you try them. If you choose to purchase, make sure that a free trial period is offered and that you can return the goods and pay nothing if they don't suit. From experience I would also advise you to get such agreements in writing before agreeing to buy!

More Information

Pain is wearing, debilitating and downright miserable. Almost all pain can be controlled, but it is only possible to do this when the doctor is told exactly how bad your pain is and what it is like (*see* Chapter 1 'How can my pain be assessed?').

Some people will not admit to pain because they are afraid of two things: either becoming addicted to their drugs, or that some day there will not be a drug strong enough to control their pain. Be assured that, when the drugs are prescribed properly, both of these fears are totally unfounded.

Chapter 5

Some questions frequently asked about pain

I have a new pain, but I am already on painkillers. What can I do?

If it is just a niggle that doesn't bother you too much or it goes away after a short time, try paracetamol, make a note and don't do anything else unless it comes back.

If it's a severe pain or is persistent, don't try adding extra tablets that were not prescribed for you. Discuss the new pain with the doctor or nurse. You might need a different type of painkiller. It might help you to look at Chapter 1 'How can my pain be assessed?'. This tells you the kind of information the doctor will need before deciding how to treat your new pain.

It might also be useful to keep a pain diary. This is described in Chapter 2 'What do I need to know about my pain?'

I have pain in my bone – how can it be treated?

Bone pain usually arises when the cancer has started to grow in a bone. This might have been picked up on an X-ray or you may be aware of pain.

Bone pain may be treated with drugs used for arthritis. You will usually be advised to continue taking morphine or another strong painkiller because often the best results are achieved by taking the two in combination.

Sometimes radiotherapy is used to help bone pain by killing the cancer cells that are causing the pain. Usually just one visit is required, but it can take several days to work, so do continue to take your painkillers exactly as you are told and don't reduce the doses until the doctor tells you to do so.

I have pain in my muscle – how can it be treated?

Muscle pain usually responds to a combination of your usual painkillers and drugs to relax the muscles given with the painkillers. Sometimes diazepam is used – so don't think it's being given to make you relax because you are too stressed. It is being used to relax your muscles but might make you slightly drowsy.

I have pain in my nerve – how can it be treated?

Pain can arise from a nerve being compressed by the tumour either pressing on it or growing into it and actually damaging it. The doctor must first decide the exact cause because they need different treatments. It is also very important for you to describe the pain as accurately as you can because this also helps to decide the best treatment. You'll find a list of descriptive words in Chapter 1, in the 'Think' section.

If your pain is coming from pressure on a nerve, steroids usually help by reducing the swelling around the nerve. You should continue to take your painkillers as prescribed by the doctor.

If the nerve is actually being damaged directly by the cancer, this can be more difficult to treat and a variety of drugs may be tried. These include medicines usually used for fits, depression or occasionally for heart problems. The reason is that these drugs help to stop the pain by affecting how the nerve functions. You'll find a bit more about this in Chapter 3 'What do I need to know about the treatment for my pain?'

I am elderly: are the painkillers safe for me?

The simple answer is, 'yes'. Most painkillers are removed from your body through the kidneys and liver. As we get older, our kidneys and liver may not be working as efficiently as they did in earlier years. The doctor may order some blood tests to check that your liver and kidneys are healthy. Older people sometimes need smaller doses of drugs.

The blood test is not a reason for you to worry; rather be reassured that the results will be used to make sure that you are given a dose of medication that is safe for you.

What is a 'pain clinic'?

It's a clinic held in some hospitals where doctors who specialise in dealing with pain see patients whose pain has been difficult to manage. If you are sent there, don't worry, it is to ensure that you are given expert advice and the specialist there will be able to advise your doctor about the treatment that is best for you.

What is a syringe driver and when is it used?

Sometimes pain is managed most effectively by injections of morphine or similar drugs. These injections need to be given every four hours, day and night, to keep pain under control. An alternative is to put a tiny needle just under your skin and attach a syringe driver.

The syringe driver is a device about the size of a personal stereo, which contains a small battery-operated motor. A syringe is attached, filled with the amount of painkiller you need for 24 hours. The syringe driver pumps a tiny amount of painkiller into your skin every few minutes. This is painless and allows you to be free from pain without having to remember to take tablets. The syringe driver can be carried in your pocket and a very long polythene tube connects it to the needle.

The syringe driver is also useful if you are having difficulty with swallowing tablets or are feeling sick.

How do skin patches work to kill pain?

Some drugs can be effectively absorbed through the skin. You may be aware of this method being used for nicotine patches to help people stop smoking, for some hormone replacement therapy and for angina.

A couple of drugs can be delivered through the skin to control severe pain. These patches are not suitable for everyone, but when they can be used, they have the advantage that the patch only needs changing every three days.

Physical Problems

Chapter 6

I've lost my appetite

The doctor says

When we are less active than normal, we use less energy, so we eat less than normal. It is also natural for people who are seriously ill to lose interest in food. Sometimes we, the patients, are less bothered about our loss of appetite than our relatives and carers. Loss of appetite usually causes our close relatives quite a bit of worry.

Cancer treatments can also reduce your appetite. This is normal and will resolve when the treatment has finished.

You might find it difficult to cope with normal flavours and textures if your mouth is sore and your sense of taste affected. This happened to me after chemotherapy and radiotherapy and I dealt with it in a rather unusual way – baby food! The jars were about the right size for my reduced appetite, the taste was fine and there were no added spices or salt to burn my raw tongue. I progressed from stage 1 to the lumpier and tastier stage 3 over a few weeks. The children had great fun teasing me about 'being in my second childhood'. This helped them cope and provided an opportunity for them to ask about my progress in a threatening situation.

We need to take time to think about what is causing the change in our appetite. That is the clue to overcoming the problem – at least in part.

Think

When did the change in appetite or loss of interest in food begin?

- Was it before this illness began?
- Was it at a time of significant change in your personal life – a change of job, retirement, or some other major event?
- Did your appetite change after you were prescribed a new medication or started on some new health product that you bought over the counter? If so, discuss this with your doctor.
- Has your weight changed significantly – a loss of more than half a stone (3 kg)?

Ask

Ask your doctor for advice about any prescribed medication that you think has made your appetite worse. There may be an alternative that will be equally effective, but that will not have this side effect. If you bought something and think it may be the cause, ask the pharmacist about it.

If your appetite still does not improve, in spite of carrying out all the advice you have been given by the nurse or doctor, ask about dietary supplements or seeing a dietician or nutritionist for further advice.

Note

Keep a note of the things that seem to help and also those that did not. Over a period of time, as different ideas are tried, it will be useful to have this record.

Your notes may also help identify any treatments that are associated with changes in your appetite or that make you feel sick.

Do

Take note of the flavours and consistency of foods that seem to suit you best. If you have a sore mouth you should avoid hard dry food and will find a soft moist diet preferable.

If your sense of taste has altered or you have difficulty in swallowing some foods, experiment and find what suits you best. Don't be afraid to try something new.

Being offered a meal that is too big for you can put you off eating. Try a smaller portion, or even a smaller plate if you wish. It is much better to finish a small portion than leave most of a larger one on the plate.

If you are eating out, don't be afraid to ask for a small portion (or even a child's portion). I did this and never once experienced any problem. The waiter or waitress has probably met someone else with the same problem. If they have not, you will be helping someone else who might ask for the same service.

Try and avoid strong cooking smells at mealtimes. Some foods (cabbage comes to mind) generate smells as they cook that can make you feel sick. If you can sit somewhere else, well away from the kitchen, that may help. Of course, it's not always possible. Try opening the kitchen window (unless it's too cold outside). If all else fails, just avoid cooking that particular food until you feel better.

By the way, adding a bay leaf to a cabbage while it is cooking eliminates the smell and does not affect the flavour.

Explore

There are various ways of ensuring that you continue to eat a reasonably good diet without having to eat 'normal-sized' meals. It is worth exploring some of these in more detail but, to get you started, a few ways to add extra calories and protein to foods are listed at the end of this chapter. There are also some tips on general ways that you might be able to improve your appetite, or at least enjoy your food a bit more. If your sense of taste has been affected by your treatment, try some of the ideas that worked for others and for me. They are also listed at the end of the chapter.

More Information

Sometimes loss of appetite can be due to other problems. These can include:

- constipation (*see* Chapter 9)
- depression (*see* Chapter 11)

- tiredness and fatigue (*see* Chapter 26)
- nausea (with or without vomiting) (*see* Chapter 21)
- painful mouth (*see* Chapter 19)
- pain elsewhere – not in the mouth (*see* Chapter 5)
- poorly fitting dentures or problems with your teeth
- treatment – chemotherapy and radiotherapy cause a temporary loss of appetite
- difficulty in swallowing (*see* Chapter 23)
- unappetising food.

If any of these problems apply to you, try and resolve the problem. It is always worth the effort.

Some ways to add extra calories and protein to your meals

- **Butter** can be added to cooked rice, cooked pasta and vegetables, etc. This adds some calories, fats and vitamins.
- **Buttering** your toast while it's hot means you get more butter and therefore more calories, fats and vitamins.
- **Creamers** (the type usually added to coffee) add calcium, glucose and vegetable fat.
- **Dried milk** added to ordinary milk (one cup per pint) doubles the protein content.
- **Mayonnaise** is fattier and has more calories than salad dressing.
- **Milk** can be used instead of water to dilute 'condensed' soups.
- **Soured cream** or cheese on potatoes adds calories and fats.
- **Sugar** can be added to cereals, or syrup to porridge, as a source of extra energy.
- **Vitamin drops** or medicines (the type usually bought for babies and very young children) may be used to provide extra vitamins. They can be added to food. Remember always to check the label and use exactly the amount recommended. Use a child's dose if you aren't sure. Cooking or heating destroys many vitamins, so the drops are best added after cooking or else added to foods not needing to be cooked.
- **Whipped cream** is full of calories and is easy to swallow. Add it to desserts and puddings.

Ice cream makers are not as expensive as they used to be. Home-made ice cream uses cream, milk and sugar – lots of fats and calories in those and you can add some pureed fruit as well.

In addition to these household ideas, there are high calorie and high protein powders which have no discernible taste. These can be added to drinks if eating solid food is difficult or when your appetite is really bad. Ask the nurse or doctor about these.

Tips for improving your appetite

- **An aperitif**, in the form of a small alcoholic drink, may help. If you are on medication, check that it is OK to have alcohol. Sometimes alcohol can interfere with the action of the medicine. Some cancer patients become intolerant of alcohol and may even experience pain after having a drink. 'Everything in moderation' is a good maxim. If you do feel unwell or experience pain after drinking even a small amount of alcohol, my personal advice is to do without the drink!
- **Cravings** for certain foods are fascinating and irritating. When I experienced food cravings, I initially tried to resist, but gradually I gave in and began to see that my body was probably in need of certain basic minerals or ingredients in those foods. As I began to recover, the cravings subsided.
- **Eat** when you are hungry. Your appetite might not be in rhythm with normal family mealtimes, but for a short spell it might suit you to eat when your body tells you to. Your appetite may be best in the morning and decrease as the day progresses. Listen to what your body says, it usually knows what it wants!
- **Exercising** before meals, if you feel up to it, will stimulate your appetite. Fresh air is an added benefit. Even a few minutes spent sitting in the fresh air can help. If you feel fit for it, it may be worth the effort.
- **Fruit juice** or lemonade stimulates the appetite. If you have a sore mouth, these might make it even more painful. If this happens, avoid all fizzy drinks. Remember, even sugar-free fizzy drinks damage your teeth!
- **Individual food preferences**, having company and where you eat can all enhance the desire to eat or drink. Eat the things you like and enjoy. If necessary, you can add a few more calories and protein by using the tips on the previous page. If you like to eat with others and enjoy company at mealtimes, try and do this, even for one meal each day.
- **Keep food out of sight** in between mealtimes. The sight of food can make you feel sick. If your appetite is poor, the sight of food can act as a constant reminder of this problem and can make you feel much worse.
- **Small portions**, attractively served, are more appetising. If eating out, most restaurants will happily serve small portions on request. Many will also omit or add a particular food on request.
- **Smells associated with cooking** can put you off eating. A small bay leaf added to the water greatly reduces the cooking smell of cabbage or sprouts during cooking . The smell of cauliflower cooking is reduced by adding lemon to the saucepan.
- **Snacks**, to nibble when you feel like it, help keep up some food intake. Grated cheese, crisps, dried fruit and nuts or yogurt are good choices.

Altered taste and loss of appetite

Chemotherapy and radiotherapy can affect how foods taste. Women who are suffering from cancer might notice that they experience the same changes in appetite and taste that they did during pregnancy.

Sometimes, simple ideas can help. The following tips might look and sound a bit odd, but be assured, they have all been used successfully.

- **During treatment**, you simply might be too tired to be bothered with cooking. If possible, try and plan ahead before starting a particularly tiring session of treatments. If you have a freezer, make sizeable quantities of dishes that can be easily thawed and heated. Freeze these in one-meal-sized portions, ready to use when you feel unable to cope with cooking. Make some a bit smaller than your usual portion in case your appetite is affected. Alternatively, a stock of 'convenience foods' and frozen meals may save you some time and effort in preparation.
- **Cold food** has less taste than warm food and is worth trying.
- **Herbal teas** can be acceptable and pleasant, taken hot or cold.
- **Mints and boiled sweets** may help if you have a bad taste in your mouth. Don't forget the increased risk of dental decay and the fact that hard sweets can cut and ulcerate your tongue and mouth, especially if your mouth is dry.
- **New flavours** are worth a try. Your tastes might have changed. Sometimes bland foods become better tolerated, especially during treatment. Radiotherapy to your head and neck can cause a sore mouth and sometimes very bland food is easiest to eat. Some types of chemotherapy can also cause a sore mouth and strong flavours and spicy foods can sting. You may not want to eat in order to avoid the discomfort, but this is not a realistic option!
- **Plastic utensils** are not only for picnics and fast food outlets! Some chemotherapy drugs can give you a metallic taste in your mouth. Using a normal metal fork or spoon can make this seem worse, but using plastic utensils may reduce this unpleasant sensation and allow you to enjoy your food better.
- **Sauces and marinades** can add moistness and flavour, both of which are lost if you have a dry mouth. Choose bland flavours if your mouth is sore.
- **Spices** can be added to disguise tastes that you are not tolerating too well, but you might be more than usually sensitive to spicy foods and they might burn your tongue.

Chapter 7

I have bad-smelling breath

The doctor says

There are lots of causes of bad breath. These range from straightforward problems that you can resolve simply to more complex reasons that might be more difficult to deal with.

Nobody wants to have bad breath. The problem is we may not be aware of it and this can be a cause for concern. Your family might not wish to say anything about it, but it is just one of those things that can happen when you're not well. If you suspect that you might have bad breath, don't be afraid to ask for an honest answer, then think about the possible causes and what you can do about it.

Think

A list of possible causes of bad breath is given below. Tick any that apply to you and take appropriate action.

Dental and mouth problems

☐ Bad breath associated with toothache, bleeding gums or sore mouth. This may be due to infection in the mouth or gums. See the dentist.

☐ Bad breath associated with denture problems. Food may be trapped under a badly fitting denture. Remove and clean your dentures after each meal. See the dentist if it does not resolve after a few days of improved hygiene.

☐ Bad breath associated with poor dental hygiene or a dirty mouth. Meticulous attention to your oral hygiene should resolve the problem.

☐ Bad breath because you have a sore mouth (*see* Chapter 19) just now and can't clean your teeth as well as usual.

Bad breath associated with food

☐ Breath that smells of garlic or onions. This is usually due to digestion of these foods and will resolve later on.

Bad breath related to illness

☐ Bad-smelling sputum (phlegm). This could be caused by a lung infection and you should ask the doctor about treatment for this.

☐ Bad breath associated with a high temperature.

☐ Breath that smells of oranges or smells sweet. This can be associated with diabetes. If you are diabetic, check your urine and blood sugar levels. If you are not known to be diabetic and the problem persists, ask the doctor for advice.

☐ Breath that smells of ammonia. This is usually due to kidney disease and you should ask the doctor for advice.

Ask

Dental and mouth problems

Ask your dentist about badly fitting dentures. Ask either the dentist or hygienist about improving your oral hygiene if you think this is the cause of bad breath. If you have toothache, see the dentist.

Bad breath associated with food

Ask your family if this is a problem for them. If it is not, continue to enjoy your spicy food or garlic if this makes food more interesting and helps you eat better.

Bad breath related to illness

If you suffer from bad breath and think that it could be associated with any of the problems listed above in the 'Think' section, ask the doctor for advice, explaining why you think you might have a problem.

Note

- Make a note of any foods that you associate with bad breath. You might wish to avoid eating these.
- Make a note of the things that help and try these again if your bad breath recurs.

Do

- Try flavoured sweets, e.g. mints, to disguise the smell of your breath – but these are not a substitute for good mouth hygiene! Use sugar-free sweets to reduce your risk of tooth decay.
- If you wear dentures, keep them well cleaned.
- Make sure you drink enough. Drinking helps to keep your mouth fresh.

Explore

I could not find anything to explore on this topic. You might find some information, but don't be tempted to spend money on products that come from dubious sources.

With respect to 'tongue cleaners' I would ask the dentist before risking hurting my tongue. A soft toothbrush is probably as good in the first instance.

More Information

If you wake up with bad breath or a sticky mouth, you might be mouth-breathing at night when you are asleep. A mouthwash of sodium bicarbonate (one teaspoon to a pint of water) loosens any sticky debris and freshens your mouth. Don't swallow this mixture. Sodium bicarbonate can make your lips a bit dry.

For more information about mouth care, *see* Chapters 18 and 19 'I have a dry mouth' and 'I have a sore mouth'.

Chapter 8

I am breathless

The doctor says

It was not until I was having my chemotherapy and was anaemic that I began to experience true shortness of breath. Only then did I feel the panic, the loss of control and inability to climb stairs or walk a reasonable distance on level ground without stopping for breath.

Shortness of breath must be one of the worst symptoms anyone can suffer. There are several possible causes for your breathlessness. Before suitable treatment can be offered to you, the doctor must identify the precise cause. For this reason, your doctor will wish to ask various questions, examine you and might order tests before deciding on the treatment best suited to you.

Patients often ask for an inhaler ('puffer') and hope this might ease their problem. In your lungs are air passages that open and close to regulate the amount of air you breathe. Tiny muscles in your breathing tubes control them. Inhalers work well when your air passages have become narrowed. Asthma makes the airways become swollen and inflamed. A steroid inhaler helps this and other inhalers can relax the muscles that constrict airways when they become narrowed. If you suffer from asthma or bronchitis, you may be using one already. If your air passages are healthy, as is the case in many cancer sufferers, then an inhaler is probably not going to help you.

If you have lung cancer and your air passage is blocked with a tumour, the inhaler will not help this problem. Inhalers help inflammation and muscle spasm in the airways but they cannot shrink tumour bulk.

The sensation of being unable to breathe adequately will often cause you tremendous panic and fear of imminent death from suffocation. Many patients have asked me if they will die during an attack of breathlessness. I had a serious chest infection and shortness of breath immediately after an operation and, one morning at around 2 a.m., when fighting to breathe I was asking myself that question too! So, I do understand the sensation and the fear, but in 25 years in medicine I have never heard of it happening.

Watching you struggling for breath will make your family feel very anxious too. They will be feeling helpless and will want to do something to make you feel better.

Think

Because shortness of breath can be associated with coughing and chest pain, you need to think about all three.

Breathlessness

- If you have ever suffered from breathlessness before, when was this? Can you relate it to an event, a new treatment or any other change?
- When do you get breathless? Is it:
  - when you exercise?
  - when you lie down?
  - when you are sitting resting?

Cough

- Do you normally suffer from a cough – including a 'smoker's cough'?
- Have you developed a cough recently? If so, when did it start?
- If you do suffer from a cough, do you normally cough up any phlegm (sputum)?
- If you do cough up phlegm, has the colour or the amount changed? Changes in sputum volume and colour all are important clues that will help the doctor decide the likely cause and choose the most suitable treatment.

Chest pain

- Have you had any pain in your chest? If so, when was the first time you had it? When do you get chest pain now? Is the pain present:
  - all the time?
  - when you exercise?
  - when you take a deep breath?
- If you are experiencing chest pain, where in your chest do you feel it?
- What is the pain like? Circle or underline a word from the following list that describes the pain best, or think of another word that describes how the pain feels. Is the pain: aching; burning; crushing; heavy; sharp; stabbing; tearing; or tight? Your description of the pain will help the doctor diagnose the cause.
- Have you, at any time, noticed any change in your colour while feeling short of breath? Have you ever had a bluish colour around your lips while feeling short of breath? If this is happening, tell the doctor about it.

Make a note of these details and discuss them with the doctor or nurse. (*See* 'Note', below.)

Ask

Ask what is the likely cause of your breathlessness. This will help you understand what your treatment is meant to do. Ask how quickly you can expect to feel relief.

If you are feeling particularly worried by your breathless attacks, or if you are anxious by nature, ask about relaxation techniques or exercises. If you suffer from panic attacks, ask about how to manage these.

Note

You basically need to make notes of the answers to the things I invited you to think about and things you might want to ask. I'll save you the bother of having to read it all again!

Do

Find a comfortable position. Most patients find that sitting reasonably upright in a comfortable chair or well propped-up in bed is best. Many people find that being at 45 degrees is quite comfortable. Lying flat may make you feel more breathless. Pillows of various shapes are available to help you sit propped up in bed or in a chair. It is worth looking for one of these.

Try these ideas to help your breathlessness. Tick the ones that you find helpful for future reference.

☐ Stop what you are doing (assuming you are doing something strenuous) and rest.

☐ Try and relax! It's easy to say, but very hard to do. Breathe slowly and steadily.

☐ Try and focus your attention on something else – not on your breathing.

☐ Be patient, the time will seem very long, but hopefully the feeling will ease soon.

☐ Don't try to hurry: when you feel ready, resume what you were doing, but slowly.

☐ Think about what will make you breathless. Pace yourself and stop for a rest before the breathlessness stops you!

☐ Eating can make you breathless. Some people find chewing exhausting. Try softer food if this is your experience.

☐ Keep your bowels regular and avoid straining when you use the toilet.

☐ Keep cool – a hot stuffy room makes your breathing feel worse. A fan or an open window can help. If you do use a fan, don't have it aimed directly at your face. Position it a little to the side so that it blows across at a slight angle. An oscillating fan, if available, is most suitable.

☐ Break your journeys into smaller manageable bits. Put a chair at the bottom of the stairs and another at the top. Sit down and get your breath before tackling the stairs and rest at the stop. Similarly, a chair mid-way between the bedroom and bathroom can be very valuable.

If you have been given any breathing exercises, practise these regularly, as instructed.

Try and relax! I know how hard this is, but your favourite music or a non-strenuous activity can help. As you relax, your sensation of breathlessness should ease. Try reading a light, easy book, solving a crossword or doing something that will help you relax and take your attention away from your breathing.

Explore

Acupuncture sometimes makes the sensation of breathlessness improve, even if lung function tests show no improvement. Forget what the tests show if you feel better! One session of acupuncture can have an effect for up to seven days. How it produces this effect is poorly understood, but it is a non-invasive treatment that you might wish to try. What is important is how you feel, not how a therapy works or what shows up on your tests!

Acupuncture might not be available in your area on the NHS and you should ask about fees before starting the treatment. It could be quite expensive and you need to know how often you might need to attend and for how long.

Some advice about finding a suitably qualified acupuncturist can be found in the 'Useful organisations' section at the end of this book. It is important to find a fully qualified and accredited practitioner.

If you are thinking about a new chair or a bed that can be adjusted to allow you to lie down or sit up, be warned – they are expensive! Make sure that you can have this type of equipment on trial, with a full refund if it doesn't suit you. Experience has taught me that such agreements should be in writing!

More Information

You might be wondering about whether oxygen would help you. The answer is that sometimes oxygen helps, but it does not help everyone. It may sound strange, but it can do more harm than good! Your body adjusts to the air you breathe according to the cause of your breathlessness. Using oxygen can make your breathing more shallow and make your *sensation* of breathlessness even worse. That's why it will probably not be offered to you.

If you have lung cancer and possess a LGV licence, ask your doctor or the DVLA about your fitness to continue driving the LGV. You should report a diagnosis of lung cancer made within the past two years and you may need to produce evidence of fitness to drive.

The DVLA web site www.dvla.gov.uk/drivers/dmed1 offers updated information about notifiable medical conditions.

Chapter 9

I am constipated

The doctor says

On our first Christmas Day together, we were living in the nineteenth century gate lodge of the hospital where I was a junior doctor. I was on duty and we decided that, since a turkey was too big for two, we'd have a tinned pheasant instead.

My wife, Alice, got a shock when she saw how much fat was in the roasting tin, so she poured it down the sink. She got a further shock when the sink blocked! In an attempt to clear it she filled the sink with water but to no avail! I eventually came home for my Christmas dinner and some unscheduled DIY!

The sink is a bit like your bowel. The problem was at the outlet which was blocked with all sorts of stuff from years of use. The congealed fat was the final straw and adding the water had no effect. The answer was to release the blockage lower down.

I achieved this by holding a large saucepan of boiling water over the 'U' bend, which was made of lead and had no trap for cleaning. The result was a huge mass of fat, bits of old mops, fibres and tea leaves and – a very freely draining sink!

The relevance of this story will be clear when you read the section 'More Information' which explains more about some of the treatments you might need.

Most of the painkilling drugs used for cancer cause constipation. In spite of having bran for breakfast and eating lots of fruit and vegetables, you almost certainly will experience some constipation. Constipation can also be due to weakness or to being less active than usual.

Strong painkillers have two effects on the bowel. Firstly, they make it slow and sluggish. Secondly, they make you lose fluid from the bowel so the motion becomes drier and harder.

The doctor will often prescribe a laxative at the same time as giving you painkillers and will ask about your bowel function. Because the painkiller has two effects on the bowel, you might need two laxatives – one to soften the motion and one to stimulate the bowel and overcome the sluggishness caused by the painkillers. Sometimes the two types of laxatives can be given as one combined medicine. If you are given two laxatives, it is essential that you take both.

Sometimes we are reluctant to talk about our bowel functions, but it is very important that the doctor knows about your problem so that you are given the correct treatment. Try and overcome your natural embarrassment: it is likely that the problem will only get worse the longer you wait. The treatment you'll need is always simplest if started early on.

Constipation is sometimes regarded as unimportant or 'normal' when we are unwell, but it makes you uncomfortable and can cause colicky abdominal pain, loss of appetite (*see* Chapter 6), nausea (*see* Chapter 21), vomiting (*see* Chapter 21), and anxiety. In elderly patients, constipation may cause confusion.

Think

The doctor or nurse might ask you what you mean when you talk about 'constipation'. This is not intended to check your understanding of the term and you should not be offended by the question. The simple fact is that what you define as 'constipation' is someone else's normal bowel habit. The nurse or doctor needs to know exactly what is 'normal' for you and how your normal bowel activity has changed.

You will probably be asked questions like these:

- What was your normal pattern of bowel action prior to your illness or starting medication?
- When did this pattern change?
- Can you associate this change with any other event, such as starting a new medication?
- When was your last bowel motion? (Or you may be asked when was your last *normal* bowel motion?)
- What was its consistency?
- Have you had any pain or bleeding?
- Have you have suffered from diarrhoea (*see* Chapter 12) or any incontinence?
- Have you bought any medicines over the counter? If so, what did you buy?

The nurse or doctor might ask about your usual diet. If there are ways of overcoming your constipation by changing your diet, these are worth trying.

One of the reasons people become constipated is because of a reduced fluid intake or increased fluid loss from the body – e.g. by sweating more than usual. Another way we can lose fluid is through vomiting (*see* Chapter 21). You will probably be asked to give an estimate of your usual daily fluid intake and might be advised to increase the amount of liquids you drink.

If you are in hospital or being cared for away from your own home, there are other issues that are worth considering with respect to the toilet arrangements. Tick the ones that apply to you.

☐	Is the toilet convenient?
☐	Is privacy adequate?
☐	Are you sharing one toilet with several other people and do you feel anxious about this?

Ask

If you are unsure, ask about how much fluid you should drink each day and how to ensure that you eat sufficient roughage.

Some laxative suspensions are very sweet. You might wish to discuss this if you do not like sweet flavours. There are some laxative powders available that are almost tasteless and can be sprinkled on food. These might be helpful if you have alteration of normal taste (*see* Chapter 6 'I've lost my appetite').

Sometimes it is necessary to use two laxatives to overcome the constipation associated with strong painkillers. You must take both, but it might be possible for you to be given a single laxative that contains both types. If you have problems with taking medicines, ask about this.

Note

Have you bought any medication over the counter or from the pharmacist? One of the commonly sold painkilling tablets is cocodamol (a combination of paracetamol and codeine) which is sold under a variety of trade names. Codeine is well known as a cause of constipation. Check and see if you have bought anything containing codeine and let the nurse or doctor know about this, or any other medication you purchased. You never know; it could be something as simple as that! Make a note of anything you buy for future reference.

Codeine is sometimes prescribed for an irritating cough. If you have been given anything for a cough, check if it contains codeine.

Make a note of any pain when passing a motion and any bleeding when you go to the toilet. Discuss these with the doctor or nurse.

Make a note of anything that applies to you from the list of things to think about.

Do

Constipation makes you miserable and it is worth trying different ways to improve your comfort while medications and other interventions are taking effect. Sometimes massage and local heat to your abdomen provide comfort, even if they don't have any effect on the constipation. Try a warm bath or a heated pad or a hot water bottle wrapped in a towel. Be very careful that you do not burn yourself – it's very easily done!

If these ideas give you some comfort, they are worth doing, but they are not a substitute for proper advice and appropriate medication.

Explore

There are lots of advertisements in the press about 'natural ways of overcoming constipation' but many of these will not be effective and some involve taking medications that could interfere with the treatment you are being prescribed.

It is probably a waste of money buying laxatives from the pharmacy. Many of the products available are not strong enough. Ask the pharmacist who deals with your prescription so that you get the best advice. You might be told to ask the doctor for advice and a prescription!

More Information

The doctor or nurse may wish to examine you. This examination could involve pressing quite firmly over your abdomen to check for areas of tenderness. This can be a little painful. It will probably be necessary to examine your back passage (rectum). This can be uncomfortable, but is important in deciding the best treatment for you.

Now it's time to read the story I told in the section 'The doctor says'. It will illustrate what I'm saying here.

If you have hard stools present in the rectum, this is usually treated by using enemas first – a small volume of fluid inserted into the back passage and sometimes left overnight to act. This may be followed by another enema of a different type the next morning. Be prepared for some discomfort and a very large result! If there is difficulty in getting a good result at home, admission to hospital for a day or so is worth the fuss and bother.

Thinking of my blocked sink and waste pipe, your back passage is like the waste pipe that I had to unblock. Giving you a laxative by mouth is a bit like adding water to the sink in that it adds more bulk above the blockage and it has nowhere to go. Once the blockage has been cleared lower down one can proceed.

After the enemas have acted, a laxative is usually given by mouth. If the laxative is given without first clearing the lower bowel, you will either develop severe crampy pain as the body tries to evacuate the hard mass of stool or will develop diarrhoea, which can be quite troublesome.

Occasionally, when there is a blockage due to hard stool higher up in the bowel, you can experience diarrhoea. This is due to the bowel content liquefying above the blockage and passing as liquid. This is why you are likely to be asked all the questions about your 'normal' bowel habit in the 'Think' section of this chapter.

If you have bowel cancer, you need to be very careful to avoid constipation. Your aim is to keep the bowel content soft. In addition to taking laxatives as prescribed, you must have a good fluid intake and avoid non-digestible foods such as fruit peel and pith because these can cause minor blockages by forming a mesh-like network in which bowel content becomes trapped.

Some practical tips follow below.

Practical tips to help avoid constipation

Constipation is almost inevitable with some of the painkillers prescribed for cancer pain unless laxatives are taken on a regular basis.

These ideas are intended to help you maintain a regular bowel action and are not intended to replace any laxatives you have been prescribed.

- **Exercise** is helpful in getting our bodies into a routine and keeping our bowels working in a regular pattern. A gentle walk should be enough and you should try and have some exercise each day if you feel well enough.
- **Fibre** (roughage) is the basic essential for our bowel function. The fibre in our food allows more bulk to form in the bowel and this leads to a more regular action. Good sources of fibre include wholewheat cereals, wholemeal bread and pasta, fresh vegetables and fresh fruit with the skin kept on. **NB** *Patients who are suffering from bowel cancer or who have a history of bowel obstruction should not eat fruit skins and pith.*
- **Grated carrot** added to soup adds colour, flavour and some fibre.

- **Fluids** are essential. Hot drinks often work best and some people find that coffee has a laxative effect. Always drink plenty of fluid if you are suffering from constipation.
- **Fruit** is helpful, especially if fresh or dried, but there is one exception. Bananas are more likely to cause constipation than relieve it. Tinned and stewed fruit is less useful than fresh fruit.
- **Home remedies** for constipation, that have been tried and proven, include prunes, prune juice and syrup of figs. Most supermarkets now stock prunes without stones, ready to eat without the need to stew them first. Prune juice is also available ready for use. This can be helpful if you don't feel like stewing your own fruit.
- **Rhubarb** is a popular home remedy for constipation. It does not work for everyone and one of the problems is that it can be very acid and sharp. The sharp, acid flavour is reduced if you stew the rhubarb in cold tea.
- **Laxatives** may be necessary if these simpler measures don't work. Ask the doctor for advice if your constipation persists.

Chapter 10

I am coughing up blood

The doctor says

It is important to note that lung cancer is not the only reason for people to cough up blood. The blood may have come from a small bleed in your stomach. This could be associated with aspirin or drugs like ibuprofen.

Of course, lung cancer is a common cause for coughing up blood. About 30% of the patients I have seen with lung cancer coughed up blood as one of their first symptoms.

In my experience, coughing up blood is always very frightening for you and your relatives. Do not feel annoyed with yourself for feeling upset by it, but do report the problem without delay.

Think

> **Tick any boxes that apply to you.**
> ☐ Have you been *coughing* small amounts of blood?
> ☐ Have you been *vomiting* small amounts of blood?
> ☐ Is your bleeding expected or 'explainable'? Do you suffer from a lung tumour, an ulcer (now, or at any time in the past), or nosebleeds?
> ☐ Are you on a drug that might cause bleeding, e.g. an anti-inflammatory such as ibuprofen or indometacin? (These are often used for arthritis or bone pain.)
> ☐ Do you suffer from any other lung or chest disease, e.g. chronic bronchitis?
> ☐ Have you had a cough with yellow or green phlegm and coughed up some blood?

Ask

If you have been started on any new treatment and started to cough up blood since it was started, ask if this could be the cause. If you suspect that the new treatment is the possible cause, ask about this.

Ask about the treatment available for you if you are coughing up blood. It may be helpful to read the next section, 'Note', first so that you have a better idea of the questions you might wish to ask.

Note

The doctor or nurse will ask about the amount of blood you are coughing up. This information helps them decide the best treatment for you. To help you understand why they might ask so many questions, here are some of the common situations that arise. You should make a note of what is happening to you.

Specks of blood in sputum (phlegm)

This might be due to a chest infection, especially if you have a cough with yellow or green sputum. You might be asked for a specimen of phlegm for the doctor to have examined by the laboratory to decide the best treatment.

If you have a dry cough (i.e. no phlegm) and coughing makes the bleeding start, you might be given something to suppress the cough. Some of these cough-suppressants can cause constipation (*see* Chapter 9).

Small globules of blood in sputum

This is usually due to a damaged blood vessel in the lung. You should report this type of bleeding quickly as there are several options for how it is best treated. Keep a detailed record of how often you cough up blood and the amount. What is most important is whether the problem is improving or getting worse.

You might be given tablets or powders to take which can help to control the bleeding.

If the bleeding does not respond to any tablets or powders prescribed, or if you are suffering from a lung tumour, the doctor might refer you to a specialist to see about the use of radiotherapy to seal the blood vessel. One treatment session is often sufficient and should be effective in a few days.

Do

- Think about the situations that seem to bring on an attack of coughing or that make you cough up blood. If exercise makes you cough, plan your activities and make sure that you get enough rest.
- If you find that certain postures or positions are more likely to make you short of breath or inclined to cough, try and find a position that eases this problem.
- Avoid things that make you cough. The ones that immediately come to mind are smoking, dust, aerosols, fumes (e.g. paint) and sudden changes of temperature – e.g. going outside after being in a warm room.
- If you know you are allergic to something that makes you cough or sneeze, try to avoid it.

Explore

The problem of coughing up blood always requires urgent orthodox medical intervention and I am personally not aware of a role for complementary therapies. I would equally advise that one does not rush into using any new 'treatment' that might be advertised which is not offered by your regular carers. I know of no herbal remedy or non-drug approach that has any proven value.

There is the question of the associated anxiety and stress, for which it might be worth exploring the role of counselling or relaxation therapy. These may be available on the NHS, but if the waiting list is too long find out about the cost of private sessions. Repeated visits could be expensive.

More Information

Frothy sputum (phlegm) with pink or brown blood can be associated with heart disease and fluid gathering in your lungs. This is often associated with shortness of breath, especially when lying flat.

A new cough with blood, which started after a period of time spent in bed, may be due to a clot in your lung. Ask the doctor for advice without delay. You may or may not also have a pain in the calf of your leg. If you do, this could be due to a clot in the leg and requires urgent medical advice.

One of the most feared possibilities is that one will have a massive bleed and die during that event. While it does happen very occasionally, it is much less common that one might think. If you are worried about this possibility, discuss it with the doctor or nurse.

If you have lung cancer and possess an LGV licence, ask your doctor or the DVLA about your fitness to continue driving the LGV. You should report a diagnosis of lung cancer made within the past two years and you may need to produce evidence of fitness to drive.

The DVLA web site www.dvla.gov.uk/drivers/dmed1 offers updated information about notifiable medical conditions.

Chapter 11

I feel depressed

The doctor says

We all vary enormously in how we feel when facing difficult times. There is no 'right' or 'wrong' way to feel or to cope with the situation we are facing. Let me outline a fairly typical response over the first few weeks.

Patients who have just been told that they have cancer commonly feel a sense of disbelief and despair and may even deny that they were told they have cancer. This usually lasts for around one week. *See* Chapter 30 'I am expecting bad news'.

For one to two weeks after being given bad news, you might experience sudden changes in your mood, fluctuating between feeling cheerful and positive, and feeling quite sad and down.

After about two or three weeks the reality of the situation has usually sunk in. By now you will probably have had more tests and will have seen other specialists who confirmed the diagnosis. At this stage you might feel ready to start 'fighting back' and may be feeling frustration over the perceived delay in starting your treatment.

It is normal to feel fear and anxiety as you face an unknown future. I had fears and I think it was worse because I knew too much and thought about things that were not really relevant to my situation! As Mark Twain said '*I have been through some terrible things in my life, some of which actually happened!*'

It's very easy to know that something can happen and then assume that it will.

I have to add that, for me, my Christian faith has been of vital importance. I believe that God will not allow anything to happen to me that is not in His plan for my life. God does not always tell us what is going on or why, but He gave me the strength to get through my first and second cancer journeys and I believe He can do so again now. I still need to plan, but I do not need to worry.

I am not alone in this thinking: the *Daily Mail* (14 August 2001)[1] reported on a research study published in the journal *Archives of Internal Medicine* showing that people with a strong faith had a better outcome to their illness.

Another paper, reviewing studies done over several decades, concludes that 'religious involvement appears to enable the sick, particularly those with serious and disabling medical illness, to cope better and experience psychological growth from their negative health experiences, rather than be defeated or overcome by them'.[2]

It's natural to feel sad when someone tells you that you have cancer. It's possibly the worst news you have ever been given. Sadness and crying are normal responses in my opinion. Fewer people than you might expect become 'clinically depressed'.

Clinical depression is a serious illness. It does not go away by itself and requires treatment from the doctor. Sadness does not respond to medication – we adjust to our new circumstances and start to live our lives again, with some changes.

It's natural to be sad if someone has told you that you have cancer, but if your sadness is making you ill, then you could be clinically depressed.

There are eight symptoms commonly associated with depression. You might wish to look at these and tick any that apply to you.

Which of these statements apply to you today?
- ☐ I feel agitated but I can't be bothered doing anything.
- ☐ I can't stop crying and feel low in my spirits.
- ☐ I feel exhausted and have no energy, but I am not on any different treatment.
- ☐ I feel less interested than usual in my normal daily activities.
- ☐ I can't concentrate on anything and I can't think properly.
- ☐ I keep thinking about death.
- ☐ My sleep pattern has changed (you could either be waking very early or sleeping much longer than usual).
- ☐ My weight has changed (you might have gained or lost weight).

How many of the boxes did you tick? To diagnose depression, usually you need to be suffering from at least five of the eight symptoms listed here. They are not all equally significant, nor are they listed in order of importance.

In other words, you can feel pretty bad, but still not be 'clinically depressed' in the medical sense of the word. You can feel awfully sad about what's happening to you and still not be clinically depressed. Taking tablets will not make you feel better if you are feeling sad and low but are not actually depressed.

You might wish to repeat this exercise and compare how you feel – hopefully you will be feeling better next time. Keep a note of your scores and the dates.

Think

There are lots of things that could be worrying you and for which help is available. Take time to think about these questions and tick any of the problems that apply.

- ☐ Activity – are you genuinely too tired, or just 'don't want to be bothered'?
- ☐ Attention span – are you more or less able to concentrate than before? Does this appear to be related to treatment you have been given?
- ☐ Memory – are you forgetting things that you really want to remember, or is it simply less threatening not to think about them?
- ☐ Mood – is your mood changing and, if so, how? Can you relate these changes to any specific events or circumstances?

☐   Pain – persistent, poorly controlled pain is very hard to bear and depressing.

☐   Personal problems – particularly when we don't have the energy to deal with them.

☐   Psychological illness or depression in the past.

☐   The future – you are probably asking, 'Is my disease curable?'

☐   Your appearance – have you lost interest in how you look and dress? Perhaps you have had disfiguring surgery and find it difficult to look at your body, or you feel unattractive. You might wish to look at Chapter 34 'I look different since my operation'.

What kinds of advice or support do you think would be helpful to you? You may need the help of more than one of these people:

- professional counsellor
- friend whom you trust, who can offer care, consolation and comfort
- minister of religion or other adviser from your particular faith
- nurse or doctor – for matters relating to your illness
- relatives who love you and care about you
- social worker – for financial and personal issues.

Ask

Do you need to ask about any of the points you ticked under 'Think'? In addition to these, are you worried about any of the following?

- Pain that can't be controlled? Look at Chapter 2 'What do I need to know about my pain?'
- The side effects of any medicines you are currently taking?
- The process of dying and what happens after death?
- Unfinished personal business?

It might help to look at some of these chapters: 'I feel like giving up' (Chapter 40), 'I want to make a will' (Chapter 44), and 'I want to think about my spiritual needs' (Chapter 43).

Don't be afraid to ask for help if you feel you need it. Asking for help and advice is not a sign of weakness or giving up. I am supposed to know a bit about suffering and illness and I'll happily admit that I asked for advice and help, partly because I needed reassurance and because it helped me to cope by talking to someone about the problem.

Note

You might find it helpful to note any of these that apply to you.

☐	Do you waken very early in the morning?
☐	How is your mood when you waken in the morning? Do you feel better or worse at the beginning of the day?
☐	How is your mood later in the day? Do you feel better or worse by evening?
☐	Do you have a low self-esteem and feel a burden of guilt? (What are you feeling guilty about? Why should you be feeling guilty?)
☐	Is your concentration bad?
☐	Do you not wish to speak to people, but just want to curl up and be left alone?
☐	Have you ever suffered from depression or a psychiatric illness?
☐	Are you having suicidal thoughts?
☐	Has anyone in your family ever been treated for depression or a psychiatric illness?
☐	Has your medication been changed recently?

Make a note of any of these that you need to discuss. They will help the doctor decide what help you need.

Do

Ask for help when you have identified the people that you think can help you. You might be surprised at the help available. For example, you do not have to be religious, or agree to a lifelong commitment to a church, before a minister will offer you support!

Talk to your family and friends. They might not fully understand how you are feeling, but do talk to them. In a sense, one has to have 'been there and done it' to appreciate how you feel, but if you don't talk to them your family will have even less of an idea of what you are going through.

Financial problems are often a major source of worry and it can be depressing trying to work out how you will cope. Talking to a social worker about it might help. There are many benefits and financial assistance available and a social worker will be able to offer up-to-date advice.

Major surgery might have left you disfigured and feeling unattractive, incomplete or 'less of a person than you were before'. It's not an easy subject to broach, but it needs to be discussed sooner or later. Look at Chapter 34 'I look different since my operation'.

Explore

Having cancer obviously affects your lifestyle for a variable amount of time. You are probably not able to work, so you have time to think – and worry! Try finding a new hobby or interest that is not too strenuous and occupies your mind and your time. Some days you will not feel like doing very much, so choose something that can be done on the days when you feel like it and left on the days when you don't.

When I was diagnosed with cancer the first time, I decided that it was time I became 'keyboard literate', so I bought a word-processor. I had been given no promises that I would recover from my illness, but I saw no point in just sitting around waiting to die! The word-processor gave me a new interest and was a bit of a challenge, but it also meant that I could start writing a letter, save it and come back to it later. Being a doctor, it also overcame the problem that nobody could read my handwritten letters anyway!

My word-processor had unforeseen advantages. When the university approached me and asked me to write some material for them, I was able to work on it as and when I felt fit and eventually send the draft scripts on a floppy disk. My word-processor had provided a new interest, a new achievement and a new career opportunity! All this because I refused to sit doing nothing and becoming even more anxious about my health!

I'm now having cancer treatment for the third time and am using my enforced time off work to finish writing this book.

More Information

By now, you will have realised that it can be very difficult to be sure whether you are suffering from sadness or clinical depression. Sometimes the doctor will suggest a trial of an antidepressant medicine to see if it helps. This can be a useful way of confirming the diagnosis of clinical depression. It may take more than two weeks for an antidepressant drug to show any benefit, so don't give up after a few days because you don't feel any better.

If an antidepressant does help, you are likely to need to take it for some time. This is because, when we are depressed, essential chemicals are lost from the brain. These chemicals control our mood and it takes a few weeks to restore adequate levels. It may then be possible to gradually reduce to a lower 'maintenance' dose provided your symptoms do not return. The maintenance dose allows your body to build up its normal supplies of the chemical and allows time for recovery.

You might need to take the antidepressant for several months to make sure you don't become depressed again. This is perfectly normal and it's much easier to continue a maintenance dose for a few weeks than go through the depression and the treatment all over again.

There are a few other things I should tell you about. Antidepressants are not intended to make you feel ecstatic and happy! The weakness, weariness and feeling generally unwell that are part of having cancer will still be there.

Some antidepressant drugs can cause nausea and vomiting (*see* Chapter 21), constipation (*see* Chapter 9) or a dry mouth (*see* Chapter 18). If these occur, do not stop the tablets, but do tell the doctor or nurse because a different medication may be available that would suit you better.

You have probably heard of St John's Wort (Hypericum). This plant has been shown to have an antidepressant action and you might be tempted to buy it because it is 'natural'. Let me warn you that St John's Wort can cause serious problems when taken with other prescribed or bought drugs. For more information about natural remedies, look at Chapter 38 'I would like to try complementary (alternative) therapy'.

References

1 Marsh B (2001) True faith really does save lives, say doctors. *Daily Mail*. 14 August 2001.
2 Koenig HG, Larson DB and Larson SS (2001) Religion and coping with serious medical illness. *Annals of Pharmacotherapeutics*. **35**(3): 352–9.

Chapter 12

I have diarrhoea

The doctor says

Diarrhoea is not usually as common as constipation among cancer patients, but there are exceptions to every rule. You can still get tummy upsets and food poisoning just like anyone else. If you are having treatment you might even be more prone to diarrhoea because your immune system is not working as well as normal. If this is the case, you will have been advised to be extra careful about cooking food thoroughly, not re-heating, avoiding fast-food restaurants and checking 'best-before dates', etc.

If you have had radiotherapy to your abdomen or pelvis, you might have some diarrhoea as a result of this treatment. The staff will have warned you about this and given advice about how long it might last.

If you have had surgery to your bowel, particularly if you have had part of the bowel removed, you might suffer from diarrhoea as a result. If you have had bowel surgery, your tolerance of various foods, especially fruit and vegetables, might have changed.

Ulcerative colitis and Crohn's disease both cause diarrhoea, but if you suffer from these diseases you will be well aware of that already.

Some medicines and tablets, including some chemotherapy drugs, can upset your tummy and cause diarrhoea. Finally, as I mention in Chapter 9 'I am constipated', severe constipation can cause diarrhoea.

Think

Think about these and answer any that apply to you.

- How long have you had diarrhoea?
- When was your last normal bowel motion?
- Had you been constipated immediately before the diarrhoea started?
- Did your diarrhoea start after starting on a new medicine or tablets?
- Have you had radiotherapy to your abdomen recently?
- Have you started taking laxatives for the first time, changed your laxative or changed the dose of your usual laxative?
- Have you eaten anything that might have upset your tummy? If anyone else in the family is affected it might be a 'tummy bug' that is responsible.
- Have you passed any mucus (slime) with the diarrhoea?
- Have you had any bleeding associated with the diarrhoea?
- Is it difficult to flush the stools away after you have used the toilet?

The doctor will use this information to decide the likely cause of your diarrhoea.

Ask

If your diarrhoea started after you were given a new tablet or medicine, ask if it might be the cause of your diarrhoea. Find out if this is a known side effect and how long it is likely to persist. An alternative treatment might be available.

If you developed diarrhoea following bowel surgery, this might be persistent. Ask about what treatment you could have to keep this problem under control. You might also want to ask about what foods to avoid, but often this is a matter of trial and error because people react quite differently to different foods.

Note

- Make a note of when you last had a normal bowel motion and how long you have had diarrhoea.
- Make a note of any changes in treatment that you think might be responsible and ask about these.
- Note any unusual or offensive smell or any change in your stool colour and tell the doctor about this.
- Keep a record of any foods that seem to upset you. In general, fruit and certain vegetables are common culprits but other foods, such as cream or a white sauce for fish, upset some people but not others.

Do

- Drink plenty of fluids to make up for the fluid you are losing from your bowels. Try and avoid fruit juices and sugary drinks as these are likely to make things worse.
- Avoid eating fruit, vegetables and high fibre foods until things settle. Re-introduce them in small portions at first, one at a time, making a note of any that don't suit you.
- If you are on a laxative, ask about reducing the dose, or even stopping it.
- Continue to take your medications as instructed and ask about any that seem to upset you.

Explore

There really is not much to explore on this topic! There are plenty of remedies that you can buy from the pharmacy for diarrhoea, but before you do buy anything tell the pharmacist what treatment you are already taking so that anything you might buy will not interfere with something you are being prescribed.

More Information 📖

The nurse or doctor will want to examine you to find the cause and decide how to treat your diarrhoea. This is likely to involve:

- an abdominal examination
- examination of your rectum (back passage) to make sure you are not constipated. If your lower bowel is congested, the stools above can liquefy and drain away as diarrhoea.

You might be asked to provide a stool sample for examination in the laboratory if a bowel infection is suspected.

Very occasionally, blood tests might be required.

Chapter 13

I have a fistula

The doctor says

A fistula is an abnormal passage or opening from one surface to another surface. They may form between two internal organs or between an internal organ and the skin surface. The word fistula comes from the Latin word for pipe or tube. Fistulas may therefore form an abnormal passage between two internal organs or may allow leakage to the outside.

Just for the record, a sinus is a cavity or hollow space. In other words, it is a blind cul de sac. It originates from the Latin word for a hollow.

Fistulas are not very common. Only about 1% of patients with advanced cancer will develop a fistula and they are commonest in bowel cancer or after radio-therapy to the pelvic area.

Basically a fistula forms either when the cancer progresses through the surface of one organ into another – e.g. from the rectum (back passage) into the vagina – or when the diseased tissues are further damaged by radiotherapy in a tumour that does not respond to this treatment.

Fistulas are very distressing but there are things that can be done to help you manage the difficulties they present.

Think

There are several problems associated with fistulas, each of which is difficult to deal with and very distressing. You might agree with some of these comments that other patients have made.

☐	The appearance of my fistula upsets me.
☐	I feel that my fistula makes me unacceptable to my partner.
☐	The fistula leaks an offensive-smelling liquid.
☐	I feel isolated because I am afraid of being socially unacceptable.

Ask

Your fistula needs to be managed according to your individual needs, so do not be afraid to ask for advice and help. Ask for a specialist nurse to see you because they have greater experience and expertise in these problems and can offer you the best advice.

If you have a fistula leaking out onto the skin, ask about absorbent dressings or whether an adhesive bag is available to absorb the leaking fluid.

If your fistula is leaking bowel content to the skin, some odour will occur. Ask what can be done to minimise it. There are several options, so do not suffer in silence.

If you develop redness or soreness of the skin, tell the nurse or doctor about these early on. There are ways of protecting your skin against the effects of being moist and becoming sore. The pain may be due to infection and, if so, this is usually easy to treat. Report the problem early because it won't get better on its own.

Note

- There are likely to be different people involved in caring for your fistula, so it might help for you to make a note of their names, what they do and how to contact them.
- Thinking of the problems you have with your fistula, make a note of the treatments and ideas that help and those that do not. This will help prevent you re-trying ideas that are not effective.

Do

Depending on the site of your fistula, there are practical ideas that might be worth trying. I have listed some of the commoner sites and some suggestions that have helped other patients.

Fistulas of the mouth

The constant leakage of saliva and of food is distressing and can affect your general health. The constant moistness may make the skin round your mouth more likely to become sore and break down.

A simple plug of clean gauze may seal off a small fistula, absorbing the excess saliva and allowing you to eat more easily.

If the constant dribbling of saliva is a problem, ask the doctor about tablets to reduce the amount of saliva you produce. You might end up with a dry mouth (*see* Chapter 18). You are the only person who can decide which is more acceptable. It's worth a try.

A fistula between the bowel and the skin surface

These can produce a large amount of fluid or more solid bowel content. Trying to contain this with a simple absorbent dressing rarely works.

A colostomy bag, fitted over the opening, may help collect the effluent when a fistula develops between the bowel and the abdominal wall. The stoma nurse will give you very valuable advice on skin protection and suggest the most appropriate bag.

If you have had a lot of surgery and have a very scarred tummy with an uneven surface, you might think that there is no way a bag will fit without leaking. Special skin fillers can be used to create a smooth even surface to overcome this problem. Ask the stoma nurse about this.

Various ideas can be tried to control odour and the stoma nurse will help you find the one that is best for you.

A fistula between the rectum and vagina

This is a very distressing problem. Talk to the nurse or doctor about whether it would help to try and make the stool firmer by:

- reducing the dose of your laxatives (if you are on a laxative)
- being prescribed something to make the stool firmer.

Vaginal tampons may also help to absorb excess fluid. Use a tampon that expands horizontally rather than vertically.

Ask the nurse or doctor about personal hygiene and reducing the risk of infection.

If you are well enough, you might be offered an operation to form a colostomy (an artificial opening for your bowel to your abdomen, with a bag to collect the bowel content). This could give you relief, but only you can decide whether you feel fit for an operation.

A fistula between the bladder and rectum

In this event, bowel content leaks into the bladder or urine leaks into the rectum. Either way, the result is very unpleasant. Surgery is the best option, if it is feasible and acceptable to you. Otherwise, attention to hygiene, and keeping the bowel content reasonably firm and manageable are the main things to do.

A fistula between the bladder and vagina

Surgery to create a urinary diversion can bring complete relief. Otherwise, try to absorb excess fluid by use of tampons and frequently emptying your bladder.

Explore

Do enquire about new techniques and treatments, but don't rush into trying anything you see advertised without asking the nurse or doctor first.

To be honest, I have not seen anything advertised that I could recommend for you to try.

More Information

Sometimes the smell of a fistula is due to infection and this can be controlled by use of antibiotics.

A variety of treatments might be discussed and this is more likely if several professionals are involved in your care. Every treatment discussed will not be suitable for you, so don't be too disappointed if ideas are suggested but not put into action. On the other hand, new treatments are becoming available all the time, so don't be afraid to ask.

Chapter 14

I have hiccups that won't stop

The doctor says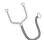

In this section, we are not thinking of the hiccups we all get occasionally, especially after a heavy meal. I am thinking of a much less common problem – hiccups that persist for hours or even days. These are exhausting and need to be treated. You probably know of several home cures for bouts of hiccups. Sadly, there is no single treatment that is consistently reliable or effective for persistent hiccups.

Think

Tick any boxes that apply to you.

☐	Did your hiccups start after changing a medication or starting a new one?
☐	Have you been under more stress than usual or upset about something recently?
☐	Have you had a recent examination involving passing a camera down your throat – e.g. an endoscopy or bronchoscopy?

Sometimes hiccups just start for no apparent reason.

Ask

If you have had any kind of endoscopy or bronchoscopy, ask the doctor if your hiccups could be related to this. Sometimes a nerve in your throat becomes irritated by the endoscope and this can cause hiccups.

If there has been any change in your tablets, ask if it could be the cause.

Note

- How long have you been hiccuping?
- Do your hiccups stop at night? You might have to ask your partner about this.
- Has the pattern of your hiccups changed – are they getting better or worse?
- Does anything seem to make the hiccups start – e.g. eating?
- If they ever stop, when is this?
- Is there a pattern to when your hiccups start or stop?

Do

Having said that treatment of hiccups can be difficult and that no single treatment can be guaranteed, there are several things that you can try yourself. These are all tried, tested and safe!

When you have tried these ideas, put a tick in the boxes beside any of the ideas that worked (even if they stop working later). This helps the doctor deduce the probable reason for your hiccups and help decide what treatments might work best.

☐ Try eating granulated sugar.
☐ Try sipping iced water or eating ice.
☐ Try sucking a fresh lemon. (Preserved lemon is not as effective for some reason.)
☐ Ask someone to massage the back of your neck.
☐ Apply ice or a cold object to the back of your neck at the level of your collar. (Put the ice inside a polythene bag to stop you getting soaked as it melts!)
☐ Try holding your breath or re-breathing into a paper bag. The hiccups should decrease, but may re-start after resuming normal breathing. If this happens, make a note and let the doctor know about it at your next appointment.
☐ Try sucking peppermints but do *not* try this if you are prescribed metoclopramide for nausea. Peppermint interferes with the action of metoclopramide.

Explore

There is an unwritten rule in medicine that the more elusive the cause, the more 'remedies' there are. Hiccups are a perfect example of this!

For this reason, you will probably come across a variety of ideas and 'cures'. Suffice it to say, if it involves taking pills or potions – don't! Before you try anything not included here, ask the nurse or doctor. Some of the items may be expensive, are a waste of money and may interfere with medicines being pre-scribed by your doctor. As I said, even simple things like peppermint can interfere with certain medicines. Ask before you try anything new.

More Information

There are many possible causes for hiccups. Don't be surprised if you are sent for blood tests to find the cause. Equally, the treatments that have been tried for hiccups are many and varied. Sometimes hiccups can be helped by medicines that are normally used for something quite different. How and why they work is not always understood. If it works for you and your doctor says it's safe to take, stop worrying and enjoy freedom from hiccups!

Chapter 15

I am itchy

The doctor says

In this chapter, we are not talking about an itchy back or leg that is helped by a good scratch! This chapter is really about itching that goes on and on, day and night and just doesn't go away. Just for completeness, a few commoner causes of itch are included.

Think

Sometimes, the cause of an itch is reasonably easy to explain and the treatment is simple. At other times it can be more difficult to find the cause and an effective treatment. Sometimes just having cancer can cause your skin to itch. The reason for this is not clear.

Itching in a small, well defined area of your body is likely to be due to a skin problem. Itching all over your body is more likely to be due to an allergy or some other internal cause. These might require treatment from the doctor or nurse.

There are many possible causes of itching, so don't panic when you read this list. Probably only one of these will apply to you. Tick anything that might apply.

Itching due to skin problems

☐	Allergy: have you been exposed to something to which you are allergic, e.g. penicillin?
☐	Contact dermatitis: a new washing powder perhaps, or starched sheets?
☐	Dry skin: especially if you are over 65. Try a moisturiser.
☐	Infestation: could you have picked up a flea from the cat or dog?
☐	Skin disease: eczema or psoriasis for example?
☐	Wet skin: have you a discharging wound or fistula (*see* Chapters 13 and 29)?

Itching due to illness

☐ Jaundice (*see* Chapter 16).

☐ Kidney problems (you will probably be aware of having a kidney problem if it is the cause): many patients on dialysis experience itching which is often worse in the summer.

☐ Lymphoma: Hodgkin's disease, or non-Hodgkin's lymphoma. (If you suffer from Hodgkin's disease, have you lost weight, had night sweats or a fever? If so, tell the doctor about these symptoms now, if you have not already done so.)

Itching due to your treatment

Has your treatment been changed recently? Radiotherapy can cause itching in the area being treated. If you are having radiotherapy, do not apply any cream to the skin without first asking for advice. Some creams can interfere with the radiotherapy treatment. For this reason, you might not be able to be offered treatment until the radiotherapy treatment has finished. Basically, many skin creams contain minute particles of metal and the metal reflects and scatters the radiation beam so that it does not reach the intended 'target'. Talcum powder can also contain metal particles, so don't use it either.

Ask

If you have ticked any of the boxes under 'Think' and have not discussed the problem with the doctor or nurse, ask for advice about these problems.

   If you are having radiotherapy, always tell the staff if you are experiencing itch or irritation of your skin. They will advise about the best treatment for you.

   I could not wait for the day when I was allowed to use a cream to cool the irritation. Cool water on a cloth helped my itch, but don't let your skin get wet for too long.

Note

Make a note of things that appear to make your itching worse or better. If you think a particular tablet or medicine might be the cause, note which medication, when you started taking it and when the itching began. The doctor or nurse will need to know all of these facts.

Do

Use a moisturiser liberally on your skin (unless you are having radiotherapy). Your skin can become very dry as a result of your illness, some kinds of treatment and from being indoors in a warm, relatively dry atmosphere.

Use a bath oil (unless you have recently had radiotherapy or have been advised not to use these products). Be careful getting into and out of the bath – you could slip easily.

Pat your skin dry rather than rubbing vigorously with a towel.

Explore

'Natural' approaches may help. For example, cucumber applied to the skin cools the skin and reduces itch. Creams based on natural plant extracts may be soothing. Always start with small amounts or ask for samples in case they don't suit you. It could become expensive otherwise!

Sodium bicarbonate (baking soda) added to a cool bath can be very soothing. Don't have the bath water too hot – that defeats the purpose!

More Information

Persistent itching is very distressing because of the loss of sleep and the sheer agony it can cause.

It can be very embarrassing to be in company and constantly needing to scratch. Try and avoid hot rooms – this makes the itch worse. Loose cool cotton clothes tend to be less irritating to your skin. I have a large selection of baggy cotton shirts as a result of my radiotherapy! They were even more comfortable after their first wash.

Don't be afraid to tell your friends that the cause of your itch is not infectious and that they won't catch it from you!

Chapter 16

I am jaundiced

The doctor says

'Jaundice' is a description, not a disease. The word is actually derived from an old French word, *jaunisse*, which means 'yellow-coloured'. At one time it was called 'the regal disease' because people believed that the only cure for it was to be touched by the king. I found no record of anyone actually being cured by this method!

Jaundice causes yellowing of the skin and the whites of the eyes, and makes you pass dark urine and pale bowel motions.

There are many possible causes for jaundice. They may be completely unrelated to your current illness. Some causes of jaundice are listed here.

- gallstones: a small stone may have got stuck in your bile duct, causing the jaundice
- hepatitis (inflammation of your liver due to infection or toxins)
- pancreatitis (inflammation of your pancreas).

Some medicines can cause jaundice, but your doctor will be aware of these and you will be told if this is the likely cause.

Think

Before you can be offered the right treatment, the exact cause of your jaundice must be correctly identified. Expect to be asked lots of questions and don't be offended if they seem inappropriate to you and your lifestyle! It's all part of the process of finding the exact cause. Alcohol abuse and infections spread by sharing needles to inject drugs are among the more common causes these days. Nobody is meaning to offend you by asking. The fact is, the doctor simply needs to know. If there is a risk of an infectious cause, blood samples are infectious too and the laboratory staff deserve to be warned.

These are the kind of questions you might be asked.

- Have you ever had a blood transfusion?
- Have you ever had jaundice before? If so, when, and how was it treated?
- Have you any pain, particularly in your upper abdomen?
- Have you suffered from itching (*see* Chapter 15)?
- How much alcohol do you drink?
- Have you ever been abroad? If so, where and when?
- Were you advised to have vaccines against hepatitis and, if so, did you have the vaccination? When?
- Had you any illness (with or without jaundice) at the time of that trip?

- Have you ever had an injection given outside the UK?
- Have you ever, at any time, given yourself an injection or shared a needle? (I know this might be an offensive question, but don't worry – I've been asked it too, as a routine question, when I was admitted to hospital.)

Ask

You will probably want to ask about the cause of your jaundice and how it can be treated.

You might wish to ask what tests are being done and how they will help the doctor who is treating your jaundice.

If you answered yes to any of the questions in the 'Think' section, you might wish to ask about these and how they might affect you now.

Note

You might want to make a note of any treatment offered and how effective it is with regard to how you feel and how it affects your jaundice.

Do

There is not a lot for you to do if you have jaundice except follow the advice you are given, get plenty of rest, eat a healthy diet, take the treatment prescribed and don't make your liver work any harder by consuming alcohol!

It's natural to worry about the medicines you are being prescribed and whether they might damage your liver. Yes, it is possible that some prescribed medications could damage your liver, but this will be carefully monitored. What is much more risky is for you to start taking other medicines or drugs as well and not telling the doctor.

Explore

On the basis of unfortunate, expensive and time-wasting experiences of others, I would advise extreme caution in exploring any course of action not recommended by your doctor.

Do not be deceived into thinking that some complementary treatments, e.g. herbal remedies, are 'harmless'. This is not always the case, as others have found out! The fact is, many are not fully researched, contain much more complex chemicals than one might think and could interfere with your medication or may be unsuitable for you.

More Information

Jaundice can be the sign of progressing disease causing increasing damage to your liver. Sometimes there is nothing that can be done to halt this process. If this is the case, which can often be determined by simple blood tests, your doctor may consider that scans and biopsies will add no new information and may not order these.

Chemotherapy and radiotherapy have been tried in the relief of jaundice. This treatment can be demanding and exhausting. Ask about how it might affect you and plan how best to cope with it.

If your disease is progressing, the changes in skin colour can develop and change very rapidly. This can be quite alarming, especially for younger members of the family.

Chapter 17

I have lymphoedema

The doctor says

Let's start with a few definitions to explain what we're talking about here.

Lymph is a fluid that is collected from the tissues throughout the body, and is returned, via the lymph nodes, to the blood. The Latin word *lympha* means 'clear spring water'.

Oedema is an accumulation of watery fluid in the tissues.

The word 'lymphoedema' is made up from these two words. Lymphoedema is the accumulation of lymph just under the surface of the skin. It causes swelling and thickening of the skin around affected areas. Usually one limb is affected, becoming swollen, heavy, tight and uncomfortable. The whole limb (arm or leg) tends to be affected.

What does lymph do?

Basically, in order to nourish the deeper tissues in our bodies, some fluid oozes out of our blood vessels, carrying food to the tissues where even the smallest blood vessels cannot reach.

After giving up nutrients, the fluid absorbs any waste products in the tissues and is reabsorbed into lymph channels and pumped back to rejoin the blood circulation so that waste products are removed. On the way back to the bloodstream, the lymph is filtered through 'lymph nodes' situated throughout your body, but especially in the groin, under the arms and in your neck. Anything that could damage the body is trapped in these lymph nodes and the body then tries to destroy the potentially damaging agent. That's why you get swollen glands during an infection – the lymph nodes are full of white blood cells which have captured germs that are being filtered out and destroyed.

What causes lymphoedema?

Lymph drains from the distant parts towards the heart, via the lymph nodes. If the lymph nodes are permanently damaged, either because they were removed, have been damaged by disease, surgery or radiotherapy, or are blocked because they have trapped cancer cells which are now growing there, the lymph can't flow freely and the affected limb swells. Usually only one side is affected.

Think

If you have lymphoedema, you are probably going to be seen by more than one professional. In making a full assessment and deciding on the best treatment for you, they will probably ask lots of questions. It might help for you to spend a few minutes thinking about how your daily life is affected by your lymphoedema.

These are the kinds of questions you might be asked. This is a long list so, I have tried to break the questions into groups.

Thinking about the timing

• How long was it, after your treatment, before you first developed lymphoedema?

Thinking about the skin around the affected area

☐ Have you any redness, heat or pain?
☐ Have you any breaks in your skin around the affected area? (A small break in the skin could allow an infection to start.)
☐ Have you had any leakage of fluid through breaks in your skin?
☐ Have you any ulcers or weeping areas on the affected skin?

Thinking about day-to-day living

☐ Do you have difficulty bending?
☐ Do you have difficulty putting on or taking off your shoes, socks, etc?
☐ Do you have difficulty with putting on clothes – e.g. fastening buttons or do your clothes become tight round your arms or legs?
☐ Is your arm or leg 'heavy'?
☐ Do you have difficulty moving around the house, climbing the stairs, or getting into bed?
☐ Can you manage to have a bath or shower?
☐ Are you at risk, e.g. when working in the kitchen? Do you suffer from cuts and grazes to the affected arm or find it difficult to hold kitchen utensils?
☐ Can you manage routine tasks unaided, or does swelling, tightness or pain in the limb stop you?

Ask

If you have ticked any of the boxes above, discuss the problem(s) you have and ask about adaptations to clothes, provision of aids to help you with daily living or with working in the house. For example, the following adaptations may help. Tick any that you wish to ask about.

☐ Long-handled devices are available to help you pick things up.

☐ Adaptations can be made to your clothes – replacing buttons with velcro and making sleeves wider and loose.

☐ Sometimes a specially designed pocket or apron can be made to support your swollen arm.

☐ Various aids are available to help you work one-handed and reduce the risk of cuts and grazes to your affected limb.

☐ If your leg is badly swollen, powered bath hoists and powered recliner/self-lift chairs can help you maintain your independence.

A physiotherapist or a lymphoedema nurse specialist may see you. They can offer a range of specialist treatments specifically suited to your needs. You might have to travel to a specialist centre to be seen.

Note

Make a note of anything that seems to make your swelling become worse or more painful. Try and avoid these activities. A similar list of the things that seem to help is equally useful.

Do

- Keep the swollen limb raised to assist drainage of fluid back into your body. Fluid always runs downhill!
- When you are resting, try and raise your arm to the height of your shoulder by using pillows or cushions. Avoid rough fabrics that could damage your skin.
- When sitting, try and keep your legs up, at least level with your hips. The foot of the bed can be raised at night by 2–3 inches. Do not use bricks, because they can slip. Specially designed 'bed-raisers' are available and must be securely fitted.
- Make sure that you *gently* exercise the affected limb 5–10 times, twice a day.
- Attend to cuts, scratches and insect bites promptly. Clean them well and apply an antiseptic cream or solution. A small cut or scratch can cause exactly the same problems as a larger one, so don't be tempted to dismiss a small injury as insignificant.
- Be very careful when cutting your toenails or fingernails. It's very easy to cut the skin, especially if it's swollen and covering the edge of the nail. If you have problems, it might be best to see the chiropodist.
- Always dry well between your fingers and toes after washing. Use a hair drier at the lowest heat setting if you have difficulty getting a towel between swollen toes or fingers or if your skin is easily damaged.
- If you develop any signs of inflammation (redness, pain or heat) ask for advice and treatment from the doctor promptly. Infection can spread rapidly and needs an antibiotic.
- Do not allow your swollen arm to be used for injections, blood samples (including finger prick samples) or blood pressure checks.
- Keep your skin in good condition and try to prevent infection. The rules are simple:
  - use a soap-free cleanser
  - dry very carefully and gently

- moisturise
- look for and report signs of infection promptly
- avoid injury – e.g. from cutting your nails, sunburn and insect bites.

Explore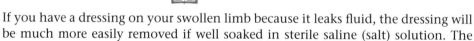

A swollen limb is unpleasant and it is tempting to seek advice via the Internet and from other sources. Having known others who have not benefited as a result of such explorations, my personal opinion is that you let your specialist carers continue their good work.

Do not buy a 'body massager' or 'intermittent compression pump' with a hollow sleeve for your arm or leg. You could do yourself a lot of harm with such a device. The advertising is often very clever, but you should only take advice from the specially trained person who has seen and assessed your limb.

Information booklets for patients with lymphoedema following treatment for breast cancer can be obtained from The Mastectomy Association of Great Britain, 26 Harrison Street, London WC1H 8JG.

If you have difficulty in obtaining the information you want, advice is also available from Macmillan CancerLine on 0808 808 2020. This line is open from Monday–Friday, 9 a.m.–6 p.m.

More Information

If you have a dressing on your swollen limb because it leaks fluid, the dressing will be much more easily removed if well soaked in sterile saline (salt) solution. The nurse will provide the sterile saline or advise you about other methods of loosening the dressing.

There are several specialist techniques used to control swelling of arms and legs. You might hear about them and wonder what is involved, so here are a few common ones. You might want to mark the ones that come up in discussion for future reference.

- **Compression bandaging**. This is a special technique involving bandaging you from fingers/toes up the whole limb. Layers of cotton wool and stretchy bandages are used to give more compression at the fingers and toes and less at the top of the limb. A specially trained nurse or physiotherapist will do this for you.
- **Compression stockings and sleeves**. These may be made-to-measure and they work by giving firm support and preventing fluid from gathering. They are designed so that the pressure is graduated, i.e. highest at the hand or foot. You should not attempt to buy your own sleeve or a 'support stocking'. Accurate measurements are the only way to ensure that you are given a properly fitted sleeve or stocking that is suited to your needs.
- **Massage**. This is certainly not the kind of massage you have after a sauna! It's a special technique, very gently massaging the tissues to encourage the lymph to flow through the swollen lymph nodes and back into the body.
- **Intermittent compression pumps**. These are of limited value. They have a role in some situations, but choosing such devices is the work of highly trained professionals. Don't even be tempted to try and choose one.

Finally, it is natural and normal to feel distress and to be upset because of your swollen deformed limb. You might wish to look at Chapter 34 'I look different since my operation'.

Chapter 18

I have a dry mouth

The doctor says

Actually, I have asked a dentist to offer input to this and the next chapter, so this section really should be headed 'The dentist says'!

Having a dry mouth is a nuisance, but there is much more to it than just nuisance value. Saliva has several functions and you need to try and replace the actions of the saliva if possible. The functions of saliva include:

- keeping our mouths moist, allowing our lips and tongue to move around without getting stuck to the roof of our mouth and our teeth. Saliva also helps to provide a slight suction, which helps to hold a denture in place
- allowing us to speak clearly (I always say that if my speech is slurred, it's because I have *not* been drinking!)
- containing calcium, which is essential for healthy teeth. The presence of saliva helps to reduce decay, especially round the margins of our gums, which become very vulnerable if our mouths are dry
- moistening and softening our food, helping us to appreciate its taste
- neutralising the acids that form in our mouths after we eat food. These acids attack the enamel surfaces of the teeth, then bacteria cause decay in the damaged surfaces
- an antiseptic action that helps to kill the bacteria that cause decay.

Think

How long you are likely to suffer from a dry mouth is important in deciding how best to manage the problem. If it is likely to last for just a few weeks, the risks to your teeth are less than if, like myself, it will be a lifelong problem. To help the dentist or doctor (and you) choose the best plan of management, you might be asked lots of questions like these. Don't panic, some of these questions won't apply to you!

- How long have you suffered from a dry mouth?
- Did it start suddenly, or develop slowly over a period of time?

Do you have other medical conditions or take any form of treatment? Tick the boxes that apply to you.

☐   Are you a diabetic? Has your control not been as good as usual recently?

☐   Have you been on any new medication? Some that may cause a dry mouth include antihistamines for allergy, anticonvulsants for fits, beta-blockers for high blood pressure, diuretics for fluid retention, some antidepressants and some strong painkillers.

☐   Have you had any kind of mouth infection recently, e.g. thrush (candida)?

☐   Have you reduced your fluid intake?

☐   Have you had radiotherapy to your head and neck?

☐   Do you need oxygen to help your breathing? Oxygen is very dry, even if bubbled through a water chamber to try and add some moisture.

☐   Have you been mouth-breathing when asleep? Yes: silly question, you don't know because you were asleep! Do you waken up with a very dry mouth, sometimes with a bad taste in your mouth? If so, you might be mouth-breathing while you sleep.

Ask

Because you lack saliva, your teeth are at risk of more rapid decay, especially round the gum margins. This raises some practical issues.

- Enquire about the use of a fluoride mouthwash.
- Ask about a fluoride gel that you can use at night when the risk is greatest. I have been using one for several years and believe it has been beneficial.
- Ask about how often you should see the dentist or hygienist. If you are prone to more rapid tooth decay, it makes sense to be seen more frequently to deal with problems early on.

Note

Some fruits are very bland and pleasant to eat. On the other hand, some that suited you when you had saliva will now be surprisingly 'sharp'. You will almost certainly have altered taste while your mouth is dry and this might change with time. Keep a note of the things you enjoy and can eat without discomfort.

Do

Make sure that you are drinking enough fluids. Your mouth can become dry if your body is even slightly dehydrated.

   Your mouth will become dry anyway, even if you are drinking plenty. Carry a small bottle of water with you and sip frequently. It feels a bit strange at first and you will get an odd glance of curiosity, but so many people carry and drink bottled water these days that you will not look out of place.

Driving can be a bit of a problem. Drinking from a bottle involves putting your head back and losing sight of the road for a moment. I overcame this by using a 'drinks holder' hung on the window of the driver's door. I also found a child's drink bottle with a plastic straw in the lid fitted perfectly. I can sip through the straw and still watch the road.

Sucking ice cubes or frozen fruit segments, e.g. orange or pineapple (fresh or tinned in natural juice – not syrup) can freshen your mouth. Pineapple is also effective in clearing away any sticky debris that gathers on your tongue. It is acidic, so have a drink of water afterwards to protect your teeth from the acid.

If you waken up with a sticky mouth, try sodium bicarbonate (1 teaspoon in a pint of warm water) as a mouthwash but *do not swallow it*. This is an excellent and cheap mouthwash when you have a sore mouth, e.g. during chemotherapy and radiotherapy. It worked very well for me.

If you develop an infection with sore or red areas, with or without white spots, see the doctor or dentist for treatment. It could be thrush infection and will not clear up on its own. If you wear dentures, keep them meticulously clean. Dentures harbour tiny particles of food and this is an ideal medium for growing infection. Remove your dentures at night unless your dentist has told you otherwise. If you wear an obturator following maxillofacial surgery, ask for specialist advice if you are having problems with recurring soreness or infection.

Pay very careful attention to your oral hygiene. If at all possible see your dentist before starting treatment such as radiotherapy to your head and neck. You probably will not want to be bothered, but it is much better to start treatment with a 'clean bill of (dental) health' and be given expert advice, than wait until you feel like it and get round to making an appointment after the treatment has finished. Any dental work you need done before starting treatment will be easier on you physically and probably cheaper!

Ask the dentist about how often you should be seen, either by a dentist or the hygienist during your treatment. You will be given good advice about any problems that might be present. Any potential problems can be dealt with before they become major issues and you will have one less thing to worry about in terms of facing long-term dental problems.

Try a small (child's) toothbrush with soft bristles. It might sound odd, but I assure you, having used one for several years now, that it is better and more effective!

Explore

If you are sensitive about drinking from a bottle of water while in public, experiment with more discreet containers. Juice bottles with an integral folding straw, like the type sold by Lakeland Plastics, are small, discreet and easy to use.

A refillable perfume atomiser is even smaller and quickly delivers moist relief with minimal intake of fluid.

Artificial saliva sprays are available too. Ask the doctor about these. Various flavoured and unflavoured formulations are available.

Various payment plans are now available to cover the rising costs of NHS or private dental care. Talk to your dentist about the availability and value of such a policy for yourself, but do check the cost of the premium.

More Information

Because you have a dry mouth, some foods can be harder to eat and even painful. Ginger nut biscuits (one of my favourites) are too hard to crunch now – they just cut my tongue. Whether at home or in company, they get dunked in my tea! Try this for hard dry biscuits and continue to enjoy them. Gravies are another way of moistening and softening food.

All forms of alcohol, including wines (red wine in particular), dry your mouth even more than usual. Cider is often suggested as a useful agent for cleaning a dirty mouth. It is excellent at removing debris, but it is very acidic and potentially damaging to your teeth.

Traditionally it has been taught that adding glycerine to water is helpful and prolongs the moistening effect. Glycerine actually dries the tissues round the mouth! My glycerine ended up being used as an anti-freeze for our pet guinea pig's water bottle!

Avoid sugary fizzy drinks. The reason for avoiding the sugary variety is obvious – the risk of tooth decay. The sugar-free drinks are also a risk for you because the carbon dioxide added to make the drink fizzy also makes it acidic, so it could be dissolving your teeth.

The traditional advice to 'suck boiled sweets to stimulate saliva' is a waste of time if your salivary glands don't work properly. It's likely that you'll just rot your teeth and give yourself painful cuts to your tongue! Sugar-free chewing gum might be more suitable, but some sugar-free sweets are very acidic, so be careful of your teeth.

On a historical note, if you suffer from a dry mouth, be thankful that you are living in the twenty-first century. We all know how our mouths go dry when we are anxious or afraid. In the Middle Ages, long before the days of the 'lie detector', this was used as a test of one's honesty! The suspect had flour put in his (or her) mouth. If 'innocent', they would produce enough saliva to allow the flour to be swallowed. A 'guilty' person's mouth would become so dry with fear that they would be unable to swallow the flour!

I wonder how many false convictions resulted from this technique? Would you be found guilty? I know I would be, and my wife says rightly so!

Chapter 19

I have a sore mouth

The doctor says

Once again, the dentist has had her say too!

Anything that makes eating or swallowing difficult for you deserves prompt attention. The staff looking after you will check your mouth regularly, but you might have pain before any visible evidence of infection can be detected. So, don't be afraid to report discomfort and try to nip any problems in the bud.

Doctors are not usually experts on dental care. While the doctor can offer a lot of good advice and treat infection if it is present, it is advisable to see your dentist or hygienist before starting your treatment, if possible. If this can be done, it means that any existing problems can be treated. If this is not feasible, do see the dentist as soon as possible after starting the treatment. I know it's the last thing you'll feel like doing, but the dentist can look, advise about hygiene and offer a wide variety of treatments for a sore mouth or any infection that might be present. Any treatment necessary can be planned and carried out when you are feeling fit to attend. The hygienist might be asked to keep an eye on your oral hygiene.

Think

There are many causes of a sore mouth. Don't panic when you read this list – many of these will not apply to you. Tick the problems that do apply to you.

☐	Are you anaemic?
☐	Are you on antibiotic treatment? This increases the risk of thrush infection.
☐	Have you got a dry mouth (*see* Chapter 18)?
☐	Have you any infection or ulcers in your mouth?
☐	Are you having chemotherapy? This can cause a sore mouth or lips, but does not always do so.
☐	Are you taking any other prescribed drugs?
☐	Do your dentures fit badly because your gums have shrunk?
☐	Have you had herpes (cold sores) following chemotherapy?
☐	Have you had recent or previous radiotherapy to your head or neck?

Ask

- If you are on antibiotic treatment, or have been recently, and developed a sore mouth following the antibiotic, ask the doctor or dentist about treatment for this.
- If you have been suffering from a dry mouth (*see* Chapter 18) and your mouth has become sore, ask for advice about the cause.
- If you have any form of mouth infection or have mouth ulcers, report these and get treatment. You will gain nothing by waiting and hoping it will go away.
- If you are on chemotherapy, you may be given treatment to prevent fungal infections, which should stop you developing thrush in your mouth. If it starts after finishing the treatment you were given, ask for advice.
- If your dentures fit badly, see the dentist.
- If you have had herpes simplex (cold sores) following chemotherapy, this can be quite persistent because your immune system may be suppressed by the treatment you had. Ask for advice if you suspect that it has recurred.
- If you are suffering from a cancer of your mouth or tongue, report any pain, especially if it has changed in any way.

Note

If you are having several treatments with chemotherapy at regular intervals, you may experience the same problems each time. Make a note of the symptoms you had and what treatments helped. Seek advice early if you suspect that the same problem is going to happen again.

Here are a few other things that might happen.

Did you notice any alteration in taste? Look at Chapter 6 'I've lost my appetite' for some ideas that might help you.

Make a note of how you most enjoyed your food. Think about:

- **temperature**: was cooler food easier to eat?
- **taste**: did you prefer foods that were more bland than usual?
- **texture**: was food easier to eat if it has been blended or minced?
- **moistness**: does it help to add gravy or a sauce?

Commercial dietary supplements such as Complan or Build-up might be easier to manage in the short term, but should not be used to replace your normal diet for any longer than necessary.

Do

Keep up excellent oral hygiene. Use a soft, small-headed toothbrush (I use a child's brush) and use a fluoride mouthwash or a fluoride gel at night. Ask your dentist about these. Some mouthwashes can sting, so try and find one that does not contain alcohol (e.g. Fluorigard made by Oral-B). I find that this one stings the least.

A home-made mouthwash, with one teaspoon of sodium bicarbonate to one pint of water, is soothing and helps clear the debris that collects in your mouth. Use it several times a day, but do not swallow it.

If you have problems with your dentures, speak to your dentist about adjusting your dentures or, if necessary, making a new set. If you are not sure about the future, a new set of dentures might be pretty low on your priority list, but you'll be able to eat better with them and a good diet is very important.

Tell the dentist what's been happening to you and show them all medication you are taking. Some drugs can affect your mouth and gums, so the dentist needs to know all the facts in order to give you the best advice.

If you gain or lose more than about a stone in weight, the shape of your mouth can also change and your dentures might need to be adjusted. If you have difficulty in attending the surgery, ask about a home visit from the dentist.

Explore

If you have financial difficulty, you should speak to your dentist confidentially about this.

More Information

When you're unwell, mouth infections become more common. When you are tired, good oral hygiene is more difficult. Dentures and toothbrushes are notorious for harbouring infection! Bacteria just love bits of food lodged around the bristles of a toothbrush and the bathroom is usually warm and moist, which bacteria thrive on.

Dentures should be brushed thoroughly – not just soaked. Toothbrushes must be replaced after you have any mouth infection otherwise there is the risk of re-infecting yourself from a contaminated toothbrush. A simple way of reducing the risk of recurring infection is to sterilise toothbrushes, bottles with integral straws, etc. with 'Milton' or baby sterilising tablets, made up to the strength recommended by the manufacturer. It has worked for me over the last nine years and we now accept the baby bottle sterilising kit as a normal part of our kitchen, even though our children are grown up!

Practical tips if your mouth is dry and sore

- **Artificial saliva**: several artificial saliva aerosol sprays, in different flavours, are available on prescription from the doctor.
- **Chilled fruit**: chilled fruit jellies, or ice lollipops, or chilled slivers of pineapple to suck (discard the residue). Tinned pineapple is easier than fresh, but do buy it in natural fruit juices, not syrup.
- **A dirty and sticky mouth** is common in the mornings. Try sodium bicarbonate mouthwashes (use 1 teaspoon in a pint of water and do not swallow the mouthwash) or try sucking pieces of tinned pineapple. Fresh pineapple can be painful on the tongue. Pineapple is acidic, so have a drink afterwards to protect your teeth.

- **When driving**, try drinking from a child's juice bottle or a sports training bottle with an integral straw. Keep it conveniently at hand in a holder for canned drinks hung on the driver's door. This avoids the need to tilt your head as you sip.
- **Good dental hygiene** is not so easy to keep up when your mouth is sore. Try a soft toothbrush to minimise trauma and ask your dentist about mouthwashes to reduce inflammation or infection.
- **Ice**: a jug of iced water or a dish of crushed ice (with a spoon) is very refreshing. Ice lasts longer than water.
- **Ice cubes** can be made from any juice or sparkling water. It makes tap water a bit more interesting!
- **Infection** is more common in a dry mouth because one of the functions of saliva is to act as an antiseptic. Dentures can cause minor injury to the mouth. This gives an excellent opportunity for infections to start.
- **Juices**: fresh orange, lemon or grapefruit juices are refreshing but these may sting your mouth. Experiment first and make a note of what you like best.
- **Mouth sprays**: a small hand-held aerosol spray filled with water or a juice of your choice can be refreshing and quite inconspicuous to use.
- **Sparkling water**: tonic or soda water is refreshing. If you wish, you could make it into home-made lollipops. Look for the lollipop moulds that allow melted ice to be sucked from the bottom of the mould (e.g. from Lakeland Plastics). This allows the option of sipping as well as sucking if your tongue is sore.
- **Sugar-free chewing gum** helps stimulate saliva.
- **The risk of decay** and the speed of tooth decay increase due to your lack of saliva. Use sodium bicarbonate mouthwash to neutralise acids in your mouth. Using a toothpaste containing sodium bicarbonate can have the same effect.

Chapter 20

I am having nightmares

The doctor says

A nightmare is an unpleasant or a frightening dream. The content of a dream or nightmare may be very significant. Sometimes you are trying to deal with fears or anxieties that you do not feel able to talk about while you are awake.

After my operation in 1994, I had a very rare reaction to a drug given to me before the anaesthetic and I stopped breathing. I was resuscitated and was in the intensive care unit.

For weeks I had the same dream – I was being given an anaesthetic and I would wake up having dreamed that I didn't wake up! By day I coped fine but at night for a spell I re-lived the experience in my dreams.

In addition to nightmares, there are other types of thoughts that we can have. Here are a few common ones.

An *illusion* is mistaking a real object or person for something or someone else. For example, mistaking a nurse for a relative.

A *hallucination* is seeing, hearing or smelling something that is not actually present. Hallucinations usually occur in the time when we are just drifting over to sleep.

Some drugs can cause hallucinations. If you think you are hearing or seeing things that are not there, tell the nurse or doctor. It is usually very easy to resolve the cause of the problem.

The doctor or nurse might explore exactly what it is you are experiencing. This is to help them decide how best to manage your problem. They are not casting doubt on what you describe. Your description plays a very important part in determining the cause and deciding the best treatment.

Think

- What are your nightmares about? Has it been the same theme night after night? Is it something that you need to talk about? If you don't feel able to discuss the problem with the family, do ask the nurse or doctor for help and advice.
- When did you start having nightmares? Was it after some significant event or a change in your medication?
- Did you like an alcoholic drink? If so, has your intake of alcohol changed? Decreasing or stopping your usual alcohol consumption can trigger nightmares. Do not be anxious about discussing this with the nurse or doctor.

Ask

If you think your nightmares are related to a change in your medicines or alcohol intake, ask about what can be done to help you not have these dreams.

Note

Make a note of when you have nightmares and of any changes to your medication and alcohol intake. This information could be very useful if the nightmares recur later on.

Do

Try to discuss any fears or anxieties you have. I had fears and anxieties too. Sometimes it is not until after the event that you realise how anxious you were! I certainly learned that knowing about cancer did not make it any easier to live with cancer. In fact, sometimes I knew too much and worried about things that really were not relevant to me. That, I suspect, is human nature, but it does not make it any less real or unpleasant when it's happening.

Explore

I would exercise caution about some of the 'techniques' and courses on offer to help one cope as these are expensive and often there are easier ways, which are also a lot cheaper.

Relaxation tapes or your favourite music may help you relax after a nightmare.

More Information

Many of the problems discussed here can be resolved by having a trusted person with whom to share your fears, feelings and anxieties. Sometimes, whether we want to admit it or not, we are actually anxious about dying. It can be frightening to think of the consequences of dying before you have finished all the things you planned to do. It can be difficult to think about the effects that your death will have on your family and friends.

Think about speaking to your minister or religious adviser. They have a lot of experience and can offer a lot of help and comfort – even if you do not go to church regularly. Perhaps you want to make peace with God. I know my personal faith has been a great source of help and comfort to me during the worst days of my three cancer journeys.

Sometimes, if all attempts to treat hallucinations and nightmares fail, the doctor may ask for the advice of a psychiatrist. Don't worry! You are not going mad! Psychiatrists are experts in understanding why our minds play tricks during illness. Why not accept expert help and get the right treatment more quickly?

Chapter 21

I am feeling sick

The doctor says

When I was having weekly chemotherapy, I felt sick every day for about three months. It is one of those symptoms that you experience, but nobody else knows just how bad it can be.

At first I was afraid to eat, but gradually, I felt more confident that I could eat and not be sick!

My nausea was always slightly worse the day *before* I was due to have my chemotherapy. Why was that? Quite simply, I believe it was anxiety about going to the hospital the next day! Yes, doctors have fears about having treatment too!

There are a number of possible causes for feeling sick (nauseated). The most effective treatment will depend on the precise cause. To determine the cause, the doctor will probably ask quite a lot of questions. It is possible for nausea to be caused by either a change in your treatment or your illness. If you suspect that your treatment is the cause, ask for advice.

While none of us likes being sick, vomiting can often relieve the sensation of nausea.

Possible causes of nausea include:

- worry, stress and anxiety, as I have already admitted
- anything that upsets your bowel function – constipation (*see* Chapter 9), indigestion or a simple tummy upset
- a build-up of chemicals in your blood due to your liver or kidneys not working as well as usual. A blood test will check if this is the reason
- almost any drug, but strong painkillers, antibiotics, and anti-cancer chemotherapy are among the common ones. Nausea associated with strong painkillers usually settles after a couple of days.

When I was a medical student, I was given a tip for the exams. I was told that if I was asked about the side effects of any drug, I could always play for time by saying 'nausea' while I racked my brain for a more specific answer!

If you are nauseated, the doctor might decide that this is a good time to review your current condition and your medication doses. This review could include a full examination and blood tests.

The doctor or nurse will explain the most likely cause of your nausea and offer advice about what is most likely to help.

Think

- When did you first start to feel sick?
- What is the pattern of the nausea? Is it intermittent or is it there all the time?

- Has this pattern changed? If it has, can you associate this change with any event?
- Is nausea accompanied by hiccuping (*see* Chapter 14) or retching?
- Has your treatment been changed? If so, try and recall when the treatment was changed and when the nausea began.
- Have you been coughing? Sometimes bad coughing bouts result in being sick.

Ask

If you can associate the onset of your nausea with any specific event, ask about this.

Ask how long your nausea is likely to last. This will help you to plan how to try and cope with it by practical measures that you can try – *see* under 'Do'.

Note

If there are lots of changes being made to your medication or you are attending for treatment, make a note of all the changes and record anything that happens in case it is related to changes in your treatment. Record anything that seems to make you feel sick and anything that helps.

If you are vomiting, make a note of the times when you are sick. This can help the doctor decide the exact cause. Do any of these apply to you?

☐	You usually vomit, with little warning, at the end of the day.
☐	You suffer from forceful vomiting early in the day.
☐	You waken with a headache and are sick.

Do

Pay attention to any dietary advice you have been given. Some of the ideas may sound terribly simple, but can be very effective.

Take any sickness medicine you were given exactly as prescribed. Even if you feel OK, your nausea might return if you stop taking it, so continue until you are told to stop.

There are a number of simple things you can try. Some may sound a bit strange, but they have been tried and they all worked for someone else. Tick the ones that help you for future reference.

☐	Avoid the smell of food cooking – especially cabbage. If you really want to cook cabbage or sprouts, a small bay leaf added to the water greatly reduces the cooking smell.
☐	The smell of cauliflower cooking is reduced by adding lemon to the saucepan (traditionally half of the 'shell' of a squeezed lemon).
☐	Let someone else do the cooking!
☐	Avoid fatty/greasy foods.
☐	Try some dry food before getting out of bed, e.g. a rich tea biscuit.

☐ After being off your food for a while, resume with clear soups, etc. and build up to 'normal food' slowly.

☐ Fizzy drinks might help – ginger/mineral water/lemonade. Taking them through a straw seems to be even more effective. I don't know why.

☐ Have drinks between meals rather than with meals.

Explore

You will find ideas in all sorts of places – old household recipe books, books of hints and tips, etc. Many are of the 'it worked for me' variety and are harmless, even if they don't work.

I would advise caution over some of the less tried and tested ideas you might come across.

You should be aware that, no matter how 'harmless' they may appear, some complementary or herbal remedies can interfere with prescribed medications. Ask the nurse or doctor before exploring the possible use of complementary therapies (*see* Chapter 38).

These complementary therapies might help and should not affect any other treatment you are being given:

• acupuncture or acupressure
• hypnosis and imagery
• relaxation techniques.

If you do decide to look further into these techniques, make sure that you consult appropriately qualified professionals. Some of these therapies are not readily available on the NHS and can be expensive.

More Information

Sometimes, when you are feeling sick, the last thing you want to do is be asked to swallow tablets. There are several ways in which anti-sickness medicine can be given. Here are some of them:

• **injections**: either repeated as required, or given in small doses via a syringe driver. When the nausea settles, you can take the tablets by mouth
• **suppositories**: inserted into the back passage
• **skin patches**: these look like a plaster for a cut, but have the medicine on a small patch and it absorbs through your skin
• **tablets that absorb** through your gums and are held in your mouth. These are not so easy to tolerate if your mouth is dry (*see* Chapter 18).

Some anti-sickness medicines can make you sleepy. This can be helpful because if you are sleepy the sickness is less likely to be so troublesome.

Sometimes your family might seem much more concerned about your vomiting than they were when you said you were feeling sick. They can see you being sick but they can't judge how bad your nausea felt. Some people find the sight of another person being sick quite alarming.

Chapter 22

I have difficulty sleeping

The doctor says

As we get older, our sleep patterns change. Many older patients have a short nap during the day and sleep less at night. This suits some people but not others. Personally, I waken up so early that I now avoid daytime napping.

Difficulty in sleeping poses major problems for some people. Sleeping tablets are not always the best solution and many doctors are reluctant to prescribe them. I have resisted any temptation to ask for sleeping tablets. My answer to the problem is to be busy by day, tired by bedtime, have a regular bedtime and to listen to relaxing music if I do waken during the night. I have a radio and CD player by my bed and a collection of relaxing CDs. I find that I often doze off again. Some mornings I am so wide awake that I won't sleep and if this is the case, I get up and do something – like writing this book!

Obviously, anxiety, fear and stress will disturb your sleep. Sleeping tablets are not going to resolve any of these.

Think

- What is your normal sleep pattern?
- When did it change?
- Can you associate this change in your sleep pattern with any event?
- What is the pattern of your sleep disturbance? Is it:
  - difficulty getting off to sleep
  - waking very early, e.g. 4 a.m.?
- Are you suffering from some physical discomfort that prevents you from sleeping? Lack of sleep can make us more aware of pain and pain interferes with our sleep. It's easy to see how a vicious cycle of events soon results.
- Are you anxious or worried about something? A similar vicious cycle may be associated with lack of sleep making you worry, and worrying leading to even more loss of sleep.
- Has there been any change in your medicines lately? Have you been in the habit of having an alcoholic drink in the evening, which you have stopped having because you are on medication?
- Are you feeling sick (*see* Chapter 21)? Nausea may prevent or disrupt sleep.
- Shortness of breath (*see* Chapter 8) can interfere with your sleep, especially if you feel that you are going to choke when you lie down.

Ask

Talk to the nurse or doctor about the pattern of your sleep and when it changed. Describe any changes in your lifestyle and ask if any of these point to a cause for the problem.

If any of the suggestions listed under 'Think' applies to you, ask the nurse or doctor about it.

Ask about any medications that you think might be causing you to sleep poorly. Some medicines can interfere with sleep. For example, if you are taking fluid tablets (diuretics) which make you need to go to the toilet, it makes sense to take these early in the day. Some others, e.g. steroids, can make you feel restless and can interfere with your sleep if you take your last dose after about 6 p.m.

Note

- There are a number of points listed under 'Think'. It might be helpful to make a note of these that affect your sleep and to record which, if any, of the ideas below under 'Do' help you to sleep better.
- Make a note of any changes to your medications that seem to affect your sleep.

Do

- Talk to the doctor or nurse about any pain you have. If you are on painkillers and are still having pain, let the doctor know.
- Caffeine is a recognised cause of insomnia, so don't have a coffee before going to bed.
- If there are any social, psychological, spiritual or financial issues worrying you, ask for the appropriate help. Your doctor or nurse can arrange for you to meet the social worker if finances are a problem. Often there are grants and other help available.
- You might want help with coming to terms with your illness, in which case counselling might help and a minister will be able to help with spiritual issues.
- Sometimes simple comfort measures are adequate. These include:
  - a hot milky bedtime drink
  - audio tapes to encourage relaxation ('relaxation tapes' are available, but sometimes your favourite relaxing music is very effective)
  - complementary therapies, e.g. aromatherapy or massage.

Explore

There are all kinds of advertisements these days for products designed to help you sleep. These range from simple products such as shaped pillows or foam mattresses to beds costing thousands of pounds.

If you do decide to buy anything very expensive like an adjustable bed, make sure you can have it on trial with a full refund if it doesn't suit you. Get any such agreements in writing!

More Information

Be wary of remedies to help you sleep that are advertised as 'natural', 'herbal' or 'homoeopathic'. These terms are not always used properly. Do not buy any of these products without first asking your doctor. Many of them, despite being described as 'safe', can interfere with tablets you might be prescribed. The product advertised may be safe on its own but in combination with other drugs, well, who knows!

Chapter 23

I have difficulty swallowing

The doctor says

Difficulty in swallowing can be caused by a number of problems. Some of these, for example thrush infection, are short-lived and will resolve quickly with treatment. Others are more serious. Whatever the cause, it can be a frightening experience if you think you are going to choke and is something you should discuss with your doctor.

Think

The doctor will ask questions about your problem. Tick the boxes that apply to you.

☐	Do you have pain when you swallow solid food?
☐	Does solid food seem to stick in your throat when you swallow?
☐	Do you have difficulty in swallowing liquids?
☐	Do you have pain when you swallow liquids?
☐	Do you suffer from a dry or sore mouth or a sore gullet?
☐	Do you have a cough, or does acid come up your throat when you lie flat?

Ask

You might already know the reason for your swallowing problem, but if not, ask the doctor about it. You might also want to ask how quickly it should resolve. This is important, because if your problem is going to persist for some time, you might need to think about obtaining items that could help, e.g. a food liquidiser.

If your problem is likely to persist for a while, you might wish to see a dietitian for expert advice.

If you have a long-term swallowing problem, ask your doctor if there are any liquid food supplements available on prescription that would be suitable for you.

Ask if any medication currently prescribed in tablet form can be given as a liquid. If this is not possible, ask which of your tablets can be crushed and swallowed with a drink.

NB: Do *not* crush any tablets without asking the doctor or pharmacist. Some are designed to act slowly over 12 or 24 hours and it is dangerous to crush, chew or try to dissolve these to make them easier to swallow.

Note

If your swallowing problem continues for some time, you might be eating less than usual. Check your weight weekly and report any significant weight loss (3 kg or half a stone) to the doctor.

Keep a record of those foods that you can swallow easily and those that cause you problems.

Do

In Chapter 6 'I've lost my appetite' there is a page giving suggestions for adding extra calories to your food. Some of these might help you maintain a reasonable energy intake while you having difficulty swallowing. Keep a note of the ideas that are helpful.

Make sure you drink enough fluids and don't become dehydrated. If you have difficulty in swallowing liquids and cannot drink as much as the nurse or doctor recommends, discuss this with them.

If you find the taste of medicines too bitter or unpalatable, try numbing your taste buds with an ice cube before swallowing the medicine. Ice cream tastes better and does the same job and also gives you a pleasant flavour to replace the unpleasant one.

Keep your mouth clean and look after your teeth. Check for redness and any sign of thrush infection (soreness and redness, possibly with white spots). If you suspect an infection or have persistent soreness, see the doctor or dentist for advice.

See the dentist if you have problems with your teeth or if you wear dentures that are causing you discomfort or don't fit well.

Check the suggestions headed 'Practical tips if you have difficulty swallowing' at the end of this chapter.

Explore

There are several different types of cup and other items available for patients with difficulty swallowing. One of these is the 'Doidy cup' – a cup that slants towards you and means that you don't have to tip your head back when you drink. These are cheap to buy and should be obtainable at larger chemists or surgical supplies stores.

More Information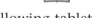

Difficulty with swallowing tablets

Some tablets can be crushed, but others must not be crushed. To be safe, do not crush anything unless you ask the doctor or pharmacist first. Some tablets are designed to be taken every 12 or 24 hours and crushing these will cause serious problems for you. Ask if it is possible for your tablets to be given as a liquid formulation.

PEG tubes

Sometimes the only realistic solution is to have a small tube inserted through the skin into the stomach. This procedure is a 'percutaneous endoscopic gastrostomy' (PEG for short) and the tube used is often called a PEG tube. Liquid food is delivered directly into your stomach via a pump. This method can be used in the long term. Because you are not drinking, your mouth may feel dry. *See* Chapter 18 'I have a dry mouth' for some practical ideas that might help.

If you have a PEG tube, you almost certainly will not be swallowing tablets. Most medicines can be supplied in liquid form or given by syringe driver if they cannot be given as liquids. *See* Chapter 5 'Some questions frequently asked about pain' for more information on syringe drivers.

If you have cancer of the oesophagus (gullet) and have a tube (stent) inserted

If you have a tube or stent inserted in your gullet you need to be careful about what you eat. The tube can become blocked with food. Your food should be soft and not at all lumpy. Avoid soft bread, stringy and pithy foods, e.g. oranges. Meat must be minced or pureed. Having a fizzy drink during and after eating helps dislodge small food particles.

If you have a tube in your gullet and food is sticking, try sipping small amounts of a fizzy drink. If this does not clear the problem and even your saliva does not go down easily, you must contact the doctor. You might need the tube to be cleared by passing a small camera to see and remove the piece of food that is causing the problem.

Practical tips if you have difficulty swallowing

- Sit in an upright position, supported by pillows if necessary.
- Keep your chin forward: this helps with the process of swallowing.
- If you are in bed, stay in a sitting position for 15 minutes after eating and drinking. This minimises the risk of heartburn and back flow from your stomach.
- Eat frequent smaller meals.
- Avoid dry and hard foods.
- Cook food until very soft and also moisten with gravy.
- Custards and jellies and ice cream can be fortified with food supplements. (Look at the page at the end of Chapter 6 'I've lost my appetite'.)
- Soup can be thickened with 'instant' dried potato powder. This adds a few extra calories too.
- Pureed food is sometimes easier to swallow than liquids – liquidise.
- A short straw requires less sucking effort than a long one. Wide-bore straws are available for liquidised food. Wide straws require less 'suck' than narrow ones.
- If you have financial difficulty and need a food blender, speak to the doctor or social worker – you may qualify for a grant.

- Try and obtain a 'Doidy cup'. This is a cup with slanting sides, available from the occupational therapist or suppliers of specialist items for disabled people. If you have difficulty in obtaining this, a 'cutaway cup' can be made from a polystyrene cup with a piece cut out for your nose, which makes it easier to swallow without tilting your head so far back.

To make a 'cutaway cup', buy some polystyrene picnic cups (the type that protect you from burning your hands). Take a sharp pair of scissors or knife and cut out a wide 'U' shape from the brim about an inch (2–3 cm) deep and the same across.

This allows you to 'raise your glass' without banging your nose on the edge. It helps you drink without tilting your head so far back. You might have to trim the cutaway portion a little to suit the size of your nose!

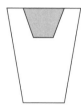

Fig. 23.1   Cutaway cup.

You may wish to contact the Macmillan Cancer Information Line on 0845 601 6161, for advice about grants and other forms of support.

Chapter 24

I am sweating

The doctor says

We all know that being in a room that is too hot will make us sweat. Sweating is one of the body's ways of cooling us down – we lose heat as the sweat evaporates from our skin.

Most of us have also experienced the sweating that is caused by anxiety, or physical distress such as pain or feeling sick.

A variety of illnesses, including some types of cancer, such as non-Hodgkin's lymphomas, can cause attacks of sweating. That's why the subject is included in this book.

Sweating causes distress and discomfort and it can be embarrassing to have to keep on wiping your brow and feeling your clothes sticking to you.

Of course, many infections also cause sweating, but this is usually associated with a raised temperature.

Think

- When did your sweating attacks start?
- Can you associate anything else with the onset of the attacks of sweating?

Ask

Ask the nurse or doctor about the likely cause of your sweating attacks. Sometimes it is possible to reduce the sweating attacks, depending on the cause.

Note

Make a note of when you get your sweating attacks. There might be a pattern, but this could easily be missed unless you keep a record of the times when they occur. This might assist the doctor in finding a suitable treatment.

Do

Simple measures can help and are worth trying. Tick the ideas that help; put a cross in the boxes beside the ideas that are less successful.

☐   Keep the room comfortably warm but not hot. You might find that a cool room is much more comfortable for you.

☐   Wear loose light clothes during the day and use cotton nightwear, bed sheets and covers. Man-made fabrics don't absorb sweat so effectively.

☐   An electric fan may help, particularly if you feel too hot. If you have a fan that moves from side to side, this is best, but if it stays in a fixed position, direct the flow of air near, but not directly at you.

☐   'Freshen up' regularly. Use cool water rather than hot. A flannel dipped in iced water, wrung out and held to your skin can be very pleasant.

☐   When you sweat, you lose quite a lot of fluid. Make sure that you have extra drinks to offset this extra loss. Cold drinks are more refreshing than hot tea or coffee.

Explore 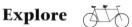

There really is not a lot to explore in terms of treatments! Excessive use of deodorants, anti-perspirants, etc. will not be very effective. The suggestions given here, along with the advice of your nurse and doctor, are the best one can offer.

More Information

Certain cancers, including lymphomas and cancer in the liver, can cause sweating attacks. This is because they produce chemicals that are released into the blood and cause you to sweat. Exactly why and how this happens is currently not well understood.

To establish the cause of your sweating, the doctor may order blood tests. These will help determine the reason for your sweating and how to treat it. It is fair to say that some of the causes remain hard to manage effectively.

Chapter 25

I have a swollen abdomen

The doctor says

As a medical student, we were taught about the causes of a swollen abdomen. Each started with the letter 'F'. The list comprised:

- **faeces**: caused by very severe constipation (*see* Chapter 9) or a bowel obstruction
- **fat**: if one is overweight or gaining weight
- **fetus**: an unborn baby (I think you would know if this is the cause!)
- **fibroids**: in the womb
- **flatus (wind)**: which would be associated with a bowel obstruction
- **fluid**: ovarian cyst or fluid collecting in the body cavity (ascites)
- **full bladder**: if there is an obstruction to passing urine.

Think

The nurse or doctor might ask several of these questions. Tick the ones that apply to you for quick reference later on.

☐	Has your waist size been increasing? Has it been measured and recorded or are you noticing clothing or belts becoming tighter?
☐	Have you been constipated? When was your last bowel motion and when did you last pass wind?
☐	When did you last pass urine?
☐	Have you been gaining weight?
☐	Have your ankles been swelling? If so, when did this start?
☐	Have you had any of the following symptoms: heartburn, acid ('waterbrash') especially when lying flat, shortness of breath on exercise or shortness of breath when you lie down? Underline any that apply.
☐	Do you need to eat less because you feel full or because you feel sick (*see* Chapter 21)?

Ask

- Ask the doctor or nurse what is causing your swollen tummy and what treatment you need.

- Ask whether the swelling will be permanently resolved by treatment or if it might recur.
- If you are having difficulty with your usual activities and normal lifestyle, ask whether there is any help available to you. Various aids and appliances are available that can assist with the activities of daily living.

Note

Is your swollen tummy affecting your daily living? Make a note of how the problem is affecting your day-to-day activities.

Any alteration in your appearance or anything that makes you look different from normal can be upsetting. Make a note of any emotional difficulties you have and discuss them with the nurse or doctor. *See* Chapter 34, 'I look different since my operation'.

Do

A swollen abdomen can make you very uncomfortable after eating. Try these ideas:

- Eat smaller meals more frequently.
- Try peppermint tea or peppermint sweets to relieve excess wind.
- If you are constipated, speak to the doctor or nurse about this.

Sometimes gentle exercise, if you feel well enough, can also help.

Report any change in your waist size or, if you have discomfort, report it to the doctor. If fluid is gathering in your abdomen, it might need to be drained.

Explore

Think about using complementary therapies to improve your mood and general comfort. Aromatherapy, massage and relaxation techniques can all help you feel better but will not deal with the cause.

More Information

Sometimes fluid tablets are used to reduce the build-up of excess fluid in your body. These do not always work, especially when the fluid is inside the abdominal cavity. The only effective way to deal with this is by draining the fluid. To do this, a small tube may be inserted under local anaesthetic and the fluid drained away over a few hours. This may be done as a day patient at hospital.

Chapter 26

I am tired all the time

The doctor says

When our son Chris was about two, I bought him a battery-operated toy drill. We always worked together on DIY projects around the house after that. One day I was putting up some shelves and ran into a problem when I found that the wall was built of stone, not brick. Chris was watching, drill in hand.

Recognising that I was having problems, Chris went to Alice who was in the next room. His message was simple: 'Too heavy.'

He returned and observed me for a couple more minutes before going back to tell his mother that it was, 'Too hard.'

After a further period of observation he announced: 'Can't do it!'

When I was having chemotherapy, I found that various items became 'too heavy', and my muscles objected to lifting shopping bags and other weighty items. Many activities became 'too hard' and, when I was too tired to be involved, I simply had to say, 'Can't do it.'

The expression 'Too heavy, too hard, can't do it' became my excuse for deferred projects and remains so to this day!

Getting down to business, there are three main questions to ask about tiredness.

- Are you having difficulty sleeping (*see* Chapter 22)?
- Are you still tired after a good night's sleep?
- Is it tiredness, or are you actually too weak (*see* Chapter 28 'I am feeling weak')?

If you are still tired after a good night's sleep, it is possible that your tiredness is due to the disease, the treatment, or the understandable anxiety you may be feeling. Feeling tired all the time may put some strain on relationships between you and your family, friends or carers. Be realistic, do what you can and, if necessary, set limits on your activity.

I used to tell patients to put a note on their front door advising callers that they were resting and did not wish to be disturbed. By setting a defined rest period each day, visitors learned when not to call. This worked for many of my patients.

Think

> Are you:
>
> ☐ Getting adequate sleep (*see* Chapter 22)? Are you sleeping enough and is it good quality sleep?
> ☐ In any discomfort or pain (*see* Chapters 1–5)?
> ☐ Anxious, worrying about something or feeling tearful and depressed (*see* Chapter 11)?
> ☐ Currently having treatment? If so, did the tiredness begin after starting treatment?

Ask

- Ask about sleep problems, but be aware that sleeping tablets are not always the answer and may make you feel even more tired and 'hung over'.
- If you have pain, even only for short periods, ask the nurse or doctor about it. There is no need for you to be in pain and the painkillers will not necessarily make you feel even more tired.
- If you are worried about something, ask for advice. It may be less of a problem than you think!
- If you feel depressed, ask for help. Depression does not go away by itself and is perfectly understandable if you are seriously ill.
- If your tiredness is due to treatment you are currently having, it should improve. Ask the nurse or doctor about when you should expect to feel better.

Note

When you are tired, you can be quite forgetful. Make a note of any things you need to do, ask or just remember. If you have a diary, this is a useful way of jotting down things that need to be done on certain days. Tick them off when you have done them, and be pleased with what you have achieved!

Make a note of anything listed under 'Think' and 'Ask' that you don't want to forget.

Keep a note of things that help you cope with your tiredness.

Do

Set realistic and achievable goals and limits for your daily activities so that you avoid getting tired through doing too much. Allow yourself time to sit and relax between the activities that you want to undertake. With regard to things that you must do each day, tackle the most physically demanding ones first when you are freshest. Start with the things you like doing least. That way, when it is later in the day and you are tired, you can look forward to doing the things that you enjoy (or at least dislike a bit less!).

Think about practical support, e.g. getting someone to help you with the more exhausting tasks in order to conserve your energy.

Be realistic about visitors! You can't always be on top of the world and, if they stay too long, they do exhaust you. If they expect a cup of tea, tell them where you keep everything and, if they offer to wash up, let them! Sometimes people *need* to be allowed to help – a lesson I only learned very late in my first illness.

Explore

There are all kinds of ideas and inventions for helping you cope when daily tasks are difficult. A few words of warning – don't spend a fortune on something 'labour-saving', only to find that in a few weeks you can manage without it. Can you borrow or hire it more cheaply?

There are lots of advertisements for vitamins, pep pills and a variety of untried, untested and unproven 'treatments' in magazines and on the Internet. However wonderful they might sound, few live up to their expectations. If you want advice about vitamins, tonics or medicine to give you more energy, ask the nurse or doctor. They may not help. One person put it quite bluntly: 'All you'll achieve is to produce expensive vitamin-enriched urine!'

More Information

Tiredness is almost always due to several factors, all going on at the same time. One possible cause is that you are anaemic. If you are attending for treatment and are having blood tests regularly, it will be picked up and treated. If you have not had a blood test for some time, discuss this with the doctor or nurse.

Before thinking about iron tablets, make sure you are eating well and drinking enough fluids. This is very important.

Radiotherapy and chemotherapy cause fatigue. It's a strange tiredness, but it does get better – I can promise you that!

I always tried to get up and show appreciation to all my visitors, even if I felt unfit. Only once did I not get up to greet a caller. I was wakened and told I had visitors but, despite my intention to get up, I fell asleep again. I felt guilty for weeks until my friends pointed out that they would have felt guilty if I had got up.

Chapter 27

I need to use the toilet, but nothing happens

The doctor says

When I was about 17, I read the story of a young nurse who lost her leg in a car crash. I was struck by her response when her boyfriend asked her one day, 'Is there anything I can do for you?' She replied, 'Go and find the leg I lost and scratch my ankle for me – it's itchy.'

After losing a part of our body, we can still feel sensations that seem to come from the part that is no longer there. These sensations appear to be generated in the brain rather than the missing body part, but they must be very distressing. They are referred to as 'phantom limb' pains or sensations.

It is also possible to suffer from a desire to go to pass water or open one's bowels, only to find that nothing happens. This ineffectual straining to do either of these is sometimes called 'tenesmus'.

This kind of problem can follow surgery or radiotherapy to the rectum, bladder or womb.

Sometimes there is pain, which may be spread over a wide area and be difficult to locate or may be very focused on a specific site. It can be caused by damage to nerves during surgery, or it may be due to nerves being trapped or damaged by a growing tumour.

Following removal of the rectum (back passage) or urinary bladder, pain and sensations of fullness can still be felt from these areas. Even knowing that this is not possible does not make the sensations any less real. One wants to use the toilet in the usual way, but logic says that this is pointless. The outcome is a very distressing problem that is extremely difficult to talk about and hard for others to understand.

Occasionally, following surgery to the bladder or womb, one has the sensation of needing to pass urine, but nothing happens. This is usually caused by damage to nerves around the bladder.

If your bladder is full, but you can't pass urine, a small tube (catheter) can be passed to relieve this. Other causes of wanting to pass urine frequently include infection or something in the bladder that is causing irritation. This could be a clot, a stone or even a catheter. These should be easy to check and deal with.

Think

☐   Have you had radiotherapy or an operation on your bladder, womb or rectum?

☐   How long have you had the feeling of needing to use the toilet? If you have been embarrassed about asking for help, try and overcome this. The problem will not settle by itself!

☐   Are you constipated (*see* Chapter 9)? Sometimes this can cause the problem or make it worse. If you have been constipated and have now developed diarrhoea, speak to the doctor or nurse and let them assess your bowels. Diarrhoea can be due to bad constipation.

If you feel the need to pass urine frequently, do any of these apply to you?

☐   Do you have difficulty completely emptying your bladder?
☐   Is it painful to pass urine?
☐   Do you pass any blood?

Ask

- If you have pain on passing urine, or are passing blood, ask the doctor or nurse about having a sample of urine checked for infection.
- If you have been constipated and have now developed diarrhoea, ask the nurse or doctor about this.
- If you have been prescribed a laxative and have developed diarrhoea since starting to take it, ask the nurse or doctor about this.

Note

Keep a note of the severity of your problem and the effects of all treatments you are given. There are several possible treatments and it helps if you keep a note of what works best for you.

Do

Make sure that you do not become constipated. Keeping your stools soft will reduce discomfort when opening your bowels and will help to ensure that you have a more effective bowel motion.

It can be embarrassing dealing with a problem such as this. To ensure that you have the time and privacy you need, invite the family to use the bathroom before you so that you do not feel anxious if you need extra time.

Simple comfort measures, such as a warm bath, may help.

Explore

This is a very distressing problem. Complementary therapies such as relaxation and aromatherapy, while they might not cure the problem, may help you to feel better in yourself. This is worth exploring.

This is a very difficult problem to treat and I am unaware of any useful treatments on offer elsewhere. My advice? Stick to the advice given by your doctor and nurse!

More Information

These problems can make you become very anxious. You are not 'weak' if you feel upset and tearful. This is a very personal problem but do not be embarrassed about discussing it with the doctor or nurse. There is always something that can be done to help you and relieve the associated stress.

Chapter 28

I am feeling weak

The doctor says

We all get tired when we have cancer and are having chemotherapy and radiotherapy. I am not talking about tiredness in this chapter but about weakness, when you find it increasingly difficult to carry out your usual daily activities.

As your disease advances, this can become quite a distressing problem. Gradually increasing weakness can become bad enough for you to spend most of your time in bed or sitting in a chair, but a sudden onset of weakness can occasionally result in your becoming completely immobile if not reported and dealt with quickly.

Think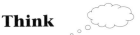

- ☐ Has your weakness come on slowly and gradually, or suddenly?
- ☐ Have you had more pain recently? Are you less active because of pain?
- ☐ Have you any back pain, loss of feeling in your feet or legs, or any difficulty passing urine? If so, report these immediately to your doctor.
- ☐ Have you had a fall recently and been weak since that event?
- ☐ Have you been feeling sad and depressed (*see* Chapter 11)?
- ☐ Has your treatment been changed recently?
- ☐ Has your blood been checked recently? If you are not eating well, you could be anaemic.

Ask

- If your weakness has come on *suddenly*, speak to the doctor *urgently*. Delays in treatment could result in permanent weakness or paralysis in some cases.
- If your pain has increased, speak to the nurse or doctor and have your pain assessed and treatment reviewed (*see* Chapter 1).
- If you have had a fall, report this to the doctor. You might have broken a bone.
- If your treatment was changed recently and your weakness came on since that change, ask the doctor or nurse if these events could be related.
- If you are feeling sad or depressed, speak to the nurse or doctor.
- Ask about a blood test if this has not been done for some time.

Note

Make a note of the time when you first felt weak, any changes that were made in your treatment just before the weakness started, and any other significant event.

Do

Try and avoid standing. A high stool might allow you to continue with some of your normal daily activities at the kitchen worktop or a table.

If you are offered physiotherapy, hydrotherapy (a bit like a swimming pool) or exercises, make every effort you can to comply with these treatments. It may be very tiring, but they can help you build up the strength in your muscles and prevent further weakness.

Continue to take all your medications as prescribed and do not stop any of your tablets unless told to do so by the nurse or doctor.

Explore

Sometimes a wheelchair can allow you to get around and get out in the fresh air. These can usually be supplied by the doctor or occupational therapist, but if there is a delay in getting a suitable wheelchair, the Red Cross might be able to lend you one. You might wish to explore this.

Find out about local taxi firms that can take wheelchair passengers and about reduced fares for disabled passengers on public transport. You can still enjoy many activities and there are hotels that have specially designed facilities for guests with disabilities.

Equipment to lift you and help you with bathing and getting into and out of bed is usually provided by the nurse or occupational therapist. The equipment should be used by trained persons. Do not attempt to buy these devices yourself.

More Information

Sudden weakness or rapidly worsening weakness, especially when associated with difficulty in passing urine, can be caused by pressure on your spinal cord. This may be due to the cancer growing and causing compression. This will not resolve by itself and requires urgent action. In the first instance you will be probably treated with high doses of steroids and might then need radiotherapy to shrink the tumour, or surgery to stabilise your spine and prevent further pressure and permanent loss of feeling and movement.

Chapter 29

I have a wound that won't heal

The doctor says

These are sometimes referred to as 'fungating wounds' because they look like certain species of fungi that have a characteristic spongy growth.

Fungating tumours, or any wound that refuses to heal, are very prone to infection. There are a number of reasons for this. The debris of dead tissue, a poor blood supply and the fact that your normal immunity is below par all contribute.

The breast is one of the commoner sites for a fungating wound to occur. Some of these are painful, particularly if infection is present, and some infections can produce quite an offensive smell. Some of these wounds do not hurt at first, but that is no reason to delay seeking medical advice.

Think

If you have a wound or any form of 'ulcer' that will not heal, think about these questions.

- How long have you had this 'ulcer'? Is it weeks, months or even longer?
- Has it ever been painful, or is the pain getting worse?
- Does it bleed, and, if so, how often?
- Is it smelly? How are you coping this problem?
- Have you ever been diagnosed with cancer? If so, how was it treated? Did you have surgery, radiotherapy, hormone therapy or chemotherapy?

If you have had cancer previously, but are not now attending for any follow-up, see your doctor without delay.

If you have not had cancer, see your doctor without delay. The chances of cure decrease with any delay in getting treatment.

Ask

Ask the doctor or nurse how your wound will be managed. It is important to be realistic about what can be done. If left too long, a wound like this might never completely heal.

Because some ulcers caused by cancer do not ever heal, goals should be realistic. The treatment you are offered will be reviewed regularly. This is not to imply that a new cure has been found, but to assess any alteration in size, colour, odour, pain, etc. and to try a different approach if necessary. Some of these are discussed here. You might wish to tick those that have been tried or make a note of things that worked for you.

Odour

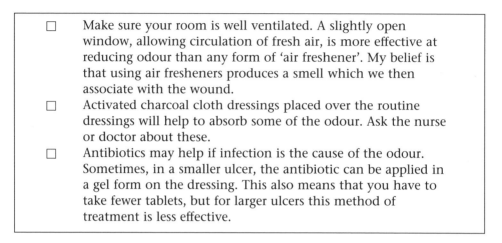

- ☐ Make sure your room is well ventilated. A slightly open window, allowing circulation of fresh air, is more effective at reducing odour than any form of 'air freshener'. My belief is that using air fresheners produces a smell which we then associate with the wound.
- ☐ Activated charcoal cloth dressings placed over the routine dressings will help to absorb some of the odour. Ask the nurse or doctor about these.
- ☐ Antibiotics may help if infection is the cause of the odour. Sometimes, in a smaller ulcer, the antibiotic can be applied in a gel form on the dressing. This also means that you have to take fewer tablets, but for larger ulcers this method of treatment is less effective.

Bleeding

- ☐ Small bleeding points can often be controlled by use of a special chemical (silver nitrate) in a small hard stick. This makes the tissue turn black, but don't panic – it's a chemical reaction, just like the tarnish on the family silver. In case you are wondering, we don't have any family silver!
- ☐ Applying a swab soaked in sodium nitrate or adrenaline (epinephrine) may control bleeding. The doctor needs to prescribe these.
- ☐ New dressings that are very effective in absorbing blood and moist secretions are appearing all the time, so ask the nurse or doctor about these.

Pain when your dressing is changed

Ask the doctor or nurse about:

- dressings that can be changed less frequently
- whether you need to take a painkiller half an hour before the dressing is changed.

Note

Keep a record of how successful the different treatments tried were for you in terms of comfort when changing the dressings and controlling the odour.

If dressing changes are painful, keep a record of the painkillers that proved most effective for you.

Do

Do not attempt to mask the smell of your wound with another odour, e.g. an air freshener or excessive use of perfume. It will not work and you will simply associate the air freshener or perfume with the wound. Soon the smell of the air freshener or perfume will become intolerable and can add to your existing problems.

Find out about dressings that absorb the odour. Ask the nurse or doctor about these.

Explore

- An operation to remove some of the unhealthy tissue may be possible in some cases. This is not a cure for the cancer but simply an attempt to reduce the size of the wound.
- Sometimes chemotherapy can result in the wound becoming smaller, even if it will not actually cure the cancer. The doctor might need to ask a specialist (oncologist) for advice about this.
- Radiotherapy can sometimes be used to reduce the size of the wound and to lessen the bleeding. Some healing may occur, which is an added bonus.
- If you are experiencing difficulties in terms of managing the problems listed above, ask if there is a specialist wound management team who could advise you.

More Information

Several drugs can be tried if there is an excessive amount of secretion from a fungating tumour. Some of these can cause drowsiness, which could be an unacceptable side effect. Ask your doctor about these if your wound is producing excessive moisture that cannot be easily managed with dressings.

The removal of an adherent dressing will almost always result in damage to the superficial blood vessels. This can also cause a variable amount of pain.

This type of wound will almost certainly affect your self-esteem. Its presence may be offensive to you and you might feel quite different about yourself. Intimacy between you and partner may be affected. Often, in my experience, we, as patients, feel much more upset about our appearance than our partners do. Don't be afraid to discuss it: how we look and feel is important. *See also* Chapter 34 'I look different since my operation'.

Personal, Social and Spiritual Problems

Chapter 30

I am expecting bad news

The doctor says

If you are facing this situation, you are facing one of the most difficult times of your life. I've been there – in the roles of giver and receiver of bad news. Let me share a few thoughts. I also suggest that you return to this chapter as often as you need to. It might help with the difficult conversations you may have to face during your illness.

From the doctor's perspective, and I speak personally here, sometimes when we give someone bad news, it 'just comes out all wrong'. Giving bad news is not easy. Sometimes we hear what we said and think, 'I didn't do that very well', but it's too late – it has been said. Be assured that no offence was intended – we've probably all said something and wished we could start all over again. The doctor may well be struggling to find the right words.

Doctors are given training in how to give bad news but, however well we plan and prepare, things don't always go according to plan. Clinics run late, things happen that should not happen, and so on.

We, the patients, recognise that the doctor is late and we think there isn't enough time to ask all the things we really need to know. We 'pick up the vibes' as we sit in a hot, crowded hospital waiting room. We watch the staff running about: we glance at the clock and the notices reminding us that clinics can run late and we sit there deciding that the burning questions in our minds will just have to wait until a less busy day.

Does this sound familiar? If it does, it's because I wrote the notes for this chapter in the hospital waiting room, as I waited to be told the news that my own cancer had recurred.

Let me offer a few thoughts that might help you during this very difficult and stressful visit to your doctor.

One criticism that has been made is that we, as doctors, try and tell our patients too much at one appointment. I know that my mind went quite blank after I heard the word 'cancer'. I was already pretty sure I had cancer, but having someone else tell you is quite different. Then it is really true! What was just a fear is now reality. It's time to re-think your whole life.

It's very hard to take the whole message on board at one appointment. By the second interview, you might be surprised at how much you apparently have forgotten. You might well ask yourself if you were actually told. You might even deny having being told some things at all. This has been proved many times by tape-recorded interviews. Patients who took the tapes home were amazed at the amount they simply didn't hear in the clinic interview. Because it was on the tape, they knew it must have been said, but they just hadn't heard.

The doctor who sees you may not know you very well. In this situation, it is hard for that doctor to estimate how much information you can handle all at once. You are also anxious about meeting someone new, what you'll be told and how you will cope with what is being said.

It's very important to hear and understand what was said and what it meant. Background noise, the strange environment, being aware of the time and talking to a complete stranger do not help. If you have any problem with your hearing or with understanding what is being said, say so! A hearing problem is nothing to be ashamed of. Too many patients smile, nod and give the impression that all is well but, in reality, they have heard very little of what has gone on. Nobody benefits – least of all you.

Think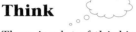

There is a lot of thinking to do here. Are you ready? Just go at your own pace and re-read this section as often as you need to – it's a good basis for any discussion where you are expecting to be given a lot of information in a short time! Here are a few of the things that will probably go through your mind.

You should try and answer each of these questions. Write the answers down if that helps. You'll probably think of other things that you want to ask about.

How much do you already know?

The important question here is what do you *know*: not what do you *think*. Is there something that you *think* might be wrong, but nobody has told you whether you are right or wrong? Find out!

Let me assure you, you are not alone if you are worrying. I worried too. All kinds of things went through my mind. The more knowledge you have, the more possibilities you'll think about.

I made a list, systematically applied my knowledge and a bit of common sense and dealt with most of my worries in that way, but I still asked a few questions to reassure myself and have someone else tell me to stop worrying.

To do this requires two things:

- the confidence that the doctor or nurse will not laugh at you (they won't)
- the guts to admit to what might seem to be a trivial or silly fear. It's still a fear, and it is not silly. If it's 'doing your head in' you need to ask!

So, don't be afraid to ask, and then either forget all about it or deal with it. I know it's threatening, but you might be worrying over nothing!

Who gave you that information?

If you do know something (in other words, you don't just think it), who told you the facts? Do you need to confirm any of the details? I am not suggesting that you seek a second opinion here, because I think there is rarely any need for this, but occasionally you might need to check that the information you have is accurate or that you have understood it properly.

How much do you want to know?

There are two ways of dealing with a difficult situation. Some people like to have all the facts and they go off and spend hours in libraries or on the Internet and explore everything in great depth. Others like the minimum of information necessary and they deal with the things they have to deal with, leaving everything else to the professionals because 'they know best'.

In the past, it was assumed that the doctor knew best. Modern medicine allows and invites the patient to be much more involved and recognises the need for knowledge and the value of working with the nurses and doctors to achieve the best outcome.

I was somewhere in the middle. I had a smattering of knowledge about cancer because I was working with cancer patients all the time, but I had never been a cancer patient myself. I found that it was easier not to grab every journal and textbook and spend hours exploring the Internet. I did not feel the need and it didn't help anyway.

I am a *patient* when I attend the clinic. I am told what I need to know and I'm invited to ask questions. I choose to be treated as a patient and, while I do ask a few technical questions, often from an academic interest, I don't request detailed information about every option available and start trying to become involved in choosing the best treatment for me. The experts decide that. I am told what they think and I go along with it.

You will be given the same opportunity to ask questions and the answers you are given will be relevant to you. That's why the person sitting next to you, with cancer affecting the same part of the body, may have been told something quite different. Cancer is a very complex illness. Your treatment is chosen to be the best for you, and exploring for detailed information, without all the specific facts relevant to each individual person, can result in your finding the wrong information.

We look again at the ways we cope with how much we need to know in Chapter 36 'I don't think my illness is as serious as they say'.

How quickly do you want to be told the news?

Doctors are advised to 'go at the pace set by the patient when giving bad news'. It's good advice. Only you know how much you can take in and how quickly it all sinks in. Do not be afraid to ask the doctor to slow down, allow you to write things down or repeat what they said, just in case you didn't hear it right.

If it's all too much too soon, say so. Ask for an opportunity to come back and hear the rest – but be aware that clinics can be booked up for some time ahead and the waiting is not easy. Your own doctor may not have all the facts at this stage either, so you can't just 'pop in and ask the GP' and expect to get all the answers.

How much do you want to be told about what is likely to happen?

The question here is basically: 'Do you want all the facts, or are you happy not to have too many specific details just now because you find that less threatening?'

There is no 'right' or 'wrong' way to do this. I have had patients who asked for all the facts 'straight from the shoulder' and others who wanted to be told very little.

We all cope in different ways. Personally I like to plan ahead, but other members of my family wait until there is some issue to deal with, then they act. At the end of the day we all achieve the same result in different ways. You must choose the method that suits you and proceed at a pace that is right for you.

You need to think about this because the staff will respect your wishes about how much you are told, but you can't blame them if something happens and you chose not to be warned that it was possible!

As well as the question of how much you *want* to know, there is the question of how much you *need* to know. None of us wants to think about the possibility of having to make a will or plan how we want our funeral conducted. The time will come eventually when we are not able to be fully involved. Someone will have to deal with these issues, so it is best for you to make your wishes known to your family, especially if you do not wish to take an active approach to your personal business at this stage.

It's OK to be silent for a few moments after being given bad news. The doctor will recognise that the message needs to 'sink in' and will go at the pace that allows you time to absorb the information you are being given.

How can you be sure you have really understood the message?

Doctors don't just use their 'medic-speak' to sound clever or confuse patients. There was a time when we might have done so. Quite simply, medical words can sum up a problem and the cause of it in a single word. We become lazy and keep our notes short by using these words. Sadly, we also cause confusion when we let them slip into our conversation with patients. If a doctor uses a word you don't understand, ask for an explanation.

There is another issue we must think about. Sometimes patients use medical terms that they have picked up during their hospital visits throughout their illness. The doctor must be sure that the patient uses these words to mean exactly the same thing as *they* mean when they use that word, otherwise confusion and misunderstanding are inevitable. So, if you feel that your understanding of a medical word is being questioned, this is why.

To try and simplify difficult concepts, the doctor may use a variety of simple terms. Commonly quoted examples include 'a shadow on your lung', 'an ulcer in your bowel that is not going to heal' or 'a wart in your bladder'.

All of these descriptions are accurate in their own right, but what do they mean to you? Don't assume that you know. Ask.

When you have been told the news, check that you understood it by telling the doctor *in your own words* what you understand to have been said. As one of my old teachers used to say, 'A parrot can recite complicated sentences, but it does not understand them!'

Do you want someone to be present with you to support you and make sure you heard everything and that you heard it correctly? Whom should you ask?

The first time I was told 'bad news', I had left my wife, Alice, in the waiting room. When I emerged, my 'stiff upper lip' gave away nothing of what had been said. We have to deal with the news eventually and sharing it early on worked for me. Alice accompanies me on all significant interviews now. She has heard things that I didn't hear because I had 'switched off'. In our discussion afterwards, we both get 'the whole message'.

The doctor may ask if you are happy for your companion to be present. This is not because they object in any way but simply because they are obliged, under laws of medical confidentiality, to check this. The information being given is confidential to you and will not be released to a third party without your consent.

If requested, a nurse can be present and she can help you afterwards with any issues that you need to re-check or clarify. She will not discuss your news with anyone else.

Ask

Having done a lot of thinking, you are probably ready to ask lots of questions.

You are allowed to ask questions! The doctor will be pleased to know that you have understood the news you have been given.

It's not always easy to ask questions just after being given bad news. Hearing it again in more detail is threatening, but what do you do a day or two later, when you are ready to talk, but your GP has not yet had a letter from the hospital specialist? This is not easy to cope with either! Ask if there is someone you can come back to speak to, for example a specialist nurse who will have access to your notes and can give you the information and support you need when you are ready.

Ask the doctor to use language that you understand. Do not be confused by any word or expression that you do not fully understand. If words like 'lump', 'tumour' or 'growth' are used, ask if these actually mean 'cancer'.

You need to remember that the doctor might not have all the information or all the results when you are seen. Doctors are fully aware of how difficult it is waiting for results and try to see you as soon as possible, but sometimes the tests take longer than anticipated to process. It can be quite difficult to get the time of the appointment right. One works on the average time taken to get similar results, but sometimes things take a bit longer. There are three questions you might wish to ask at this stage.

- Have you got all my test results now?
- Do I need any more tests to get the final diagnosis and decide the best treatment?
- If the results are not available or more tests are needed, when are you likely to have these and be able to give me a firm diagnosis and a plan for my treatment?

Note

Make a note of anything that you want to ask about.

You will be asked questions about your present illness, your past health and illnesses and any medicines, etc. that you are taking. It might be helpful to jot down some facts beforehand. I can assure you that my mind went blank! That's rather embarrassing for a doctor! I now take my notes in my pocket. I bring my medical history summary and my reminder note of things to discuss. If you are taking any medication, bring it with you. It's easier to hand over the bottles and boxes than try and remember all the complicated names, strengths and the times when you take everything.

Do

You might find it helpful to bring a pen and some paper with you. I am not suggesting that there is time to sit writing down every word that is said, but a few key words might be useful. I used to write down the main messages for my patients if they asked me to do so. A few words can act as a memory-jogger later.

You might also find it helpful to make a note of the important questions you have. Try not to bring a 'shopping list', but if you really must do so be prepared to be asked to make a longer appointment at a later date. I know the waiting is agony, but it is quite impossible to offer every patient a lot of extra time in a busy clinic. With adequate warning, the staff will do their best to give you the time you need. Deal with the main issues now and negotiate a suitable time for a longer discussion.

Explore

It is quite likely that, a couple of days after your first appointment, you will have questions that you want answered. Recognising that it takes a few days for letters to be typed and sent back to your family doctor, you might wish to explore these issues.

- Do you need to make another appointment to discuss anything – e.g. more results?
- Who else could offer advice? Is there a specialist nurse that could help? Will they have access to your notes and the relevant details?

As you sit at home over the next day or two, you will be thinking about the news you have been given. You will probably be asking yourself the following questions.

- Have you been given all the information you want or need (assuming it is currently available)?
- Did you understand what was said?
- Did you ask about who is available to offer support and clarify what you discussed?

If the answer to any of these is 'no', make a note of the things you need to ask at your next appointment.

More Information

Giving a patient bad news is one of the hardest things a doctor has to do. Usually it is a meeting between two complete strangers, in unfamiliar circumstances and at a very stressful time. It's hard to 'get it right'. The other thing is, no matter how skilfully it is done, bad news cannot be turned into good news.

The doctor's aim in this 'bad news' appointment is to:

- explore what you know about your illness
- inform you about your illness, your individual treatment plan and the likely outcome of your treatment
- answer your questions about your illness, the treatment and the longer-term outlook. Remember, things can change.

One interview won't always achieve all these aims unless it is very long or is recorded on a tape for you to listen to later. At such a stressful time, often quite soon after an operation or other investigations, you may not be at your best for taking it all on board. A second interview or an appointment with your GP is often necessary to clarify details.

Chapter 31

How do I tell my children the bad news?

The doctor says

This is another very difficult situation to handle and how you do it depends partly on the age and the understanding of the children concerned. What you tell them and how you tell them should reflect their age and ability to take in what you are saying.

Children differ in their maturity, understanding and experience, so every child needs to be assessed and treated according to their individual circumstances and ability.

Do not bypass a younger child and speak only to the older one. Do not ignore all the children and speak only to the adults. Children see, hear and sense things. They are curious by nature and will be asking questions, even if they have not uttered a single word. The impressions created now will last for a very long time, so be prepared to give the same message, clearly, simply, accurately and repeatedly for some time until the child is able to come to terms with a constantly changing and threatening situation.

The following guide may help you in assessing how much your child might understand. They are all very different and this is only a rough guide.

Ages 0–5

At this age, the concept of time is poorly developed and one toddler may think that a minute without its mother is an intolerably long time. Another will play happily, apparently oblivious to a half-hour passing. So it is with the concept of death separating them from a parent permanently. They often have not got the ability to comprehend this concept.

What is often more frightening is simply the fact that a parent is not there. It's the fact that they are absent now, not the length of the absence, that matters to this age group.

Ages 6–10

By this age, a sense of 'forever' increasingly develops. These children are still very dependent on others and will feel very vulnerable if their security is threatened. Loss of a parent or their disappearance 'forever' is very threatening.

This age group has the ability to think about the future and is used to anticipating and making simple plans for a medium-term future. Their focus, however, is usually more on the present.

Ages 10–teens

By this stage, the concepts of time, permanence, failed aspirations, hopes and dreams are increasingly established and understood.

This is the age where the child might feel cheated, angry and resentful, sometimes focusing on the loss of opportunities that *they* would have had if the patient had not developed their illness.

Think

What ages are the children who need to be told your news?
What does the child already know?

In Chapter 30 'I am expecting bad news', we looked at the concept of you thinking about what you already know before the 'bad news interview'. It is exactly the same for a child. Do you know what they actually know or are you assuming that you know? Who told them what they 'know'? If nobody has actually spoken to the children, assume that they have not got the right facts and start from that point.

What does the child actually understand?

This is not quite the same as the previous question. It is a mixture of what they can be expected to understand, based on age, individual ability and experience, and making sure that, if they have overheard adult conversations about the illness, they have not misunderstood or misinterpreted what was said. Children are children, not miniature adults.

Have the children had any warning that they might be given bad news?

If you have been attending the doctor, felt unwell, been off work or suffering for a while, the children may be aware that something is not right. They might have said nothing, but don't assume that means they were not wondering and probably discussing it among themselves.

Use this situation to establish common ground for your discussion. Introduce the idea that you have been to the doctor because you are not well and build on these familiar concepts to introduce the more serious message.

Have they had any previous experience of illness or death?

In my case, my father-in-law died four weeks before my diagnosis. Our children, then aged ten and eight, knew he had died of cancer. My concern was that they might reasonably think that everyone suffering from cancer would die soon. They were unaware of the years of good health Grandad had enjoyed since his initial diagnosis and treatment. To them, he was well and able to play with them, then suddenly he went into hospital and died a few weeks later.

Such an experience is bound to influence a child. How did we handle it?

While I was in hospital, actually the day after I was told I had cancer, Alice took Chris and Sharon into our garden. She asked them what colour the trees were. Thankfully they were evergreen conifers, because it was February!

'Green,' they replied.

'Are they all the same shade of green?'

'No.'

Using this analogy, Alice explained that the word 'green' describes a number of different shades of the same colour. In the same way, the word 'cancer' describes a number of diseases, which can behave quite differently.

When they came to see me that night, the children said, 'So you might not die like Grandad did, even though you have cancer too?'

We took it that they had understood Alice's message. They certainly asked lots of questions. We answered each question honestly and at a level appropriate to their knowledge and understanding.

Ask

There are questions you might wish to ask yourself and your spouse or partner, your children and others.

Ask yourself

Which one of us is going to tell the children?

We decided that Alice should do this because we agreed on the concept of the colour of the trees to explain how there are different types of cancers and that it was not always a 'death sentence'.

Having agreed that Alice would speak to them, we also knew that they would be back to visit me that evening and I would follow up the conversation with them. We did not want them to think that they could or should only ask Mum and not Dad. We told them that they could ask anything they wanted to know and that we would always tell them – even if it was bad news.

They said that this was what they wanted us to do.

Where should we tell them?

It is best to try and find a quiet place for such a discussion. Children are probably best to hear this kind of news at home, where their bedroom and a favourite toy are available, if they want privacy and time alone to think and come to terms with what they have just been told.

When do we tell them?

We had a dilemma. I was in hospital, so should Alice tell the children now or wait until I was home and we could talk to them together?

We decided that, because it was likely that I would have visitors who were doctors and nurses, Chris and Sharon might overhear something. We agreed that we should tell them first. So, Alice told them our news, at home, between afternoon and evening visits to see me. I spoke to them later in the ward.

There are no right or wrong answers to these questions, but I felt less stress when I knew that we could all talk openly as a family about my test results, treatment plans and how my illness might affect our family life and holiday plans.

Why wait? What's to be gained? You might not have all the answers now. That needn't be a problem. Just explain that you don't have the answers, but when you have the answer, you'll tell them. Children worry too – and worrying over something small is just as stressful as worrying over something big. Finding the answer can give the child a lot of relief and even comfort.

It won't be the first time if your child asks a question that you didn't think to ask, but it may be a question that you need answered too!

Ask your children

Obviously what you ask your children depends on their age and individual ability.

What do they know?

As always, these conversations must start on 'common ground'. Don't assume that they *know* anything. They might think they know, but they could have misunderstood.

Gently explore what they think is wrong, what it means and how it affects them and you. Be prepared for the focus of their thoughts to be on how it affects them. This is not selfish – it is normal for a younger child. They are threatened by the uncertainty of something that is going on, over which they have absolutely no control.

Having found out what they think is happening, correct any misunderstandings and tell them the truth, simply, clearly and honestly. Be prepared to do this several times.

If appropriate, ask where they heard anything that is seriously inaccurate.

Ask others

It's not easy telling your children that you have a serious illness. If you feel that you cannot cope with this task, ask the doctors or nurses if there are trained staff who can help you.

Note

Make a note of what you told the children. If the illness is likely to be prolonged, it can be difficult to remember what you discussed and when. Keeping a note can act as a useful memory-jogger later. It also allows you to correct anything that changes, e.g. when your treatment plan has been changed and you have to cancel or postpone a planned activity. Such a note can help with the 'But you promised . . .' response which is to be expected from a disappointed child.

Do

Do not force a child to listen or do something they do not want to do

If your child is not ready to listen, you can do more harm than good by forcing them to listen or talk. Tell them that when they are ready to talk, you will be there for them and make sure they feel secure in your love and care.

If appropriate, gently tell them that asking others might result in their being given the wrong information.

An older child might ask for the facts to be written down, to be read in privacy, in their own time. If this is requested, make sure that you also reassure them that you are there for them when they are ready to talk.

Keep the discussion short and focused

To keep you focused, a list of facts you need to share might help. If you are asked for it, hand it over.

Don't overload the children by saying too much too fast. Small amounts of information at a time are all that a child can be expected to take on board. Be prepared to repeat it several times, to let the child take it all in.

Include them in what is going on

Keep the children up-to-date with significant developments and events, but expect some blank silent stares in response. If necessary, check that they heard. They usually did. If you fail to keep them updated because they fail to respond, you'll only add to your own stress.

Expect a response

It may be a silent one!

Keep a list of resources and help available

When you hear a good idea, see a book that helped, or you speak to someone who can offer useful practical advice, keep a note of these useful resources. You might need them later on.

Tell the school

Teachers are trained in helping children who are facing problems and difficulties. Young children often ask teachers for support and help. Letting the teacher know the facts empowers them to correct misunderstandings, help the child prepare for difficult times and also helps explain any behavioural problems, lapses in concentration or poor performance.

Examination boards are very sympathetic to how examination performance can be affected by having a seriously ill parent or sibling. Telling the school is not 'asking for special treatment'. It is simply allowing the examiners the opportunity to assess a pupil's standard of work throughout the year, not just a performance over a few hours at a time of intense stress and poor sleep.

Make time for the children

You are facing a very busy time, possibly visiting hospital, facing extra washing and ironing, etc. and I am saying you need to make more time for the children!

It's not a case of spending lots of time together: they'll know you are unwell. Try and pay attention to them when you are with them. Focus on them specifically at family mealtimes and other times together.

Check that they understood your message

Check that they understood what you said by encouraging them to tell you what is happening *in their own words*.

Explore

There are several books and helpful guides available to help children understand about illness, death and dying. Some of them might be helpful but I suggest that you spend a while browsing through the content and how well they suit your needs.

I found the following titles in a Christian bookshop and they might be helpful.

- *My grandma has gone to Heaven*[1] is written for children aged 5–8 and points to God as a source of strength and comfort in this difficult time. It deals with that anger and confusion a young child may feel at such times.
- *Alice's Dad*[2] is a book for grieving children who are a bit older. In a separate section there are notes on each of the chapters explaining more about various aspects of illness and death (including murder and suicide), bad news, weight loss, funerals, etc.
- *You'll never believe what they told me*[3] is a book by children with cancer, for children with cancer. These children share their faith in God and how that faith helped them cope.

My local library suggested three other titles. These were:

- *Helping children cope with grief* by Rosemary Wells (1988)
- *Helping children with ill or disabled parents* by Julia Segal (1996)
- *What do we tell the children?* by Kirsten Phillips (1996).

Sadly, they did not have copies of any of these so I have not been able to peruse the contents, but most bookshops will have a selection of books on this topic.

More Information

Children need to feel secure. One issue that might be causing anxiety concerns who will look after them if a parent dies. Obviously, this is a difficult question to raise, so it might help if you introduce it first.

If there are insurance policies that will pay off outstanding mortgages and allow for a steady income to the remaining parent so that they need not work full time, share this information simply and reassure the child that they are still secure and, most of all, loved.

Young children may be afraid that their parent's illness is in some way their fault. This unfounded fear is something I have come across and it needs to be explored and addressed.

References

1   Foxhall AS (1998) *My grandma has gone to Heaven*. Christian Art Publishers, Vereeniging.
2   Merrington B (1999) *Alice's Dad*. Kevin Mayhew Ltd, Suffolk.
3   Dockrey E and Dockrey K (1994) *You'll never believe what they told me*. Chariot Books, Illinois, USA.

Chapter 32

How do I tell others the bad news?

The doctor says

If you think that I am about to write you some kind of 'prescription' telling you what to do, think again!

There is no formula that I know of and no protocol to follow. You must decide what is right for you, your family, friends and others who need to know.

I will try and offer some ideas and things to think about and share what I did.

On the first day when I was told I had cancer, I saw the consultant at 11 a.m. I went straight back to work, met with the senior staff, told them I had cancer and that I would be 'off work until I was back'. That was easy because I was working in a hospice where 90% of our patients had cancer. Everyone understood the situation.

I also told the senior staff to tell everyone the truth and that there was to be no secrecy or partial truth-telling. I followed this up with an open letter to all the staff within a few days.

Arriving home, while Alice packed my suitcase for me to be back in hospital by 2 p.m., I phoned my parents and my brother. We were living in Scotland: they were in Northern Ireland, so we could not avoid a difficult phone call. Before you think, 'But you have done it before', let me say that it never gets any easier and all I could do was try and be calm and very clear in my message.

I recognised that I had left my elderly parents and my brother devastated by what they had just heard. There was nothing I could do. What were the choices? Should I have told them a half-truth and left Alice to explain the rest later? Should I only have told my brother (also a doctor) and left him to pass on my news to my parents in person? Why did I do what I did?

As I sat in the clinic, the doctor asked me what I thought was wrong with me. I heard myself say that I thought it was cancer. I was aware that it was my voice speaking and suddenly it all sank in – this is about me. This is not about someone else sitting in a clinic on the other side of the desk or in a bed. I have cancer. Much as I want to run away, I must take this on board, face facts and act accordingly. I saw it as my personal responsibility.

Recognising that I did not want to believe it, nobody else wanted to believe it either. It is not something people want to hear, but it seemed best that I told them the truth, making no differences on the basis of age or position, except where it was appropriate to simplify the message, as for our young children. I discussed telling the children in Chapter 31 'How do I tell my children the bad news?'

Think

The situation you are facing affects you the most, but it also affects other people.

Your family, friends and work colleagues will all be affected in different ways by your illness. Plans for holidays, retirement, a wedding or other significant event may suddenly change.

Apart from yourself, who is affected by your current circumstances? In the early stages, you can't plan too far ahead and you are probably too numb to even think about it in any detail. I can assure you that you will probably not think of everything at once, so be prepared to repeat this exercise soon and every time your circumstances change significantly.

Think about yourself. How does this illness affect:

- your family?
- your friends?
- your home life and plans?
- the plans you had for the immediate and longer-term future?
- your spouse or partner?
- your work?
- you – in any other aspect of your life not included above.

Ask

There are things you need to ask yourself and there are things you might need to ask others about.

Firstly, you need to ask yourself how you wish to handle the following issues.

- Who needs to know?
- Why do they need to know?
- What do they need to know?
- When do they need to know?
- How do I tell them?
- Where should they be told?

Who needs to know?

Because I was working in a hospice, I decided that everyone at work needed to know what was happening. I included patients in this list. Does that sound strange? It was actually a good thing that I did tell patients, for I met several in the hospital clinics later on!

A couple of patients whom I had visited at home took a few minutes to recognise me in my new role. Some expressed surprise seeing me sitting among them because I was 'just another patient'. It was a strange experience, but I was exactly that – a patient – and that's what I am now. I just happen to have some experience of also being a doctor.

Who needs to know about your current circumstances? It's probably family, friends and work colleagues that will make up most of the list, but what about those policies you signed up for years ago and have forgotten all about, for example:

- insurance policies – e.g. permanent health insurance, holidays, income protection

- mortgage protection plans
- payment protection plans to cover hire purchase, etc.

Take time to go through your files and papers. You might be well rewarded for your forward planning!

Why do they need to know?

Some people need to know what's happening so they can plan ahead. If you will be off work for six months, can your employer offer a fixed-term temporary contract to someone who can do some of your work while you get on with your treatment? It does take some pressure off your mind if you can discuss these things with your employer and be involved in the planning process – if you wish to be so involved.

Your family needs to know what is going on if they are going to be involved in your life or your day-to-day care. If they had plans for a holiday or some event that coincides with a time when they might wish to be available to offer you support, then the opportunity to re-schedule might be advantageous to both parties.

I think family members should also be told simply because they are your family. It's pretty hurtful to hear this kind of news 'secondhand', but I am well aware that 'Happy Families' is sometimes only a card game for children.

Which of your friends needs to know is obviously a matter of personal choice. In our case, we included the news in a letter with our Christmas cards. Close friends whom we saw more often had heard already, but this way nobody was left out. News travels pretty fast and, in my case, our minister announced my news in the church (with my consent) and many local friends heard that way. There is always the risk that news is misunderstood or misreported which brings us to the next point.

What do they need to know?

Put simply, they need to know the truth, in as much detail as is appropriate. If you decide to 'edit' your message or give slightly varied versions to one person or another for whatever reason, you can run into problems. You'll need to remember what you said and to whom. Why should you make your life even more complicated? There is nothing to be ashamed of in being ill.

Obviously, there are certain details that do not need to be shared with everyone. If you have breast cancer, your work colleagues do not need to know whether you just had the lump removed, had a breast reconstruction or a mastectomy. By the time you return to work they should not be aware of what was done because you should be looking and feeling well.

In such cases, where information is more sensitive and personal, make sure you keep a note of what details you have decided to release to individuals. Make sure that you ask them to respect your privacy.

I found it easiest to tell the truth. The amount of detail you offer can be tailored to individual understanding on a 'need to know' basis. For one person it's enough to say that you are having treatment for three months. Another might need to be aware that you attend hospital regularly and can't drive yourself. Friends drove me to and from hospital daily for five weeks. Others were unaware of this and didn't need to know.

Then there is the issue of claims and insurance policies. Every company from whom you are entitled to make a claim will want certified evidence of the nature of your illness, etc. They will possibly ask for private certificates or send reports for your GP to complete and sign. There is a fee payable for this service, so be aware of this and also keep records of all visits to your GP and clinic appointments.

When do they need to know?

With respect to your family, they probably know something anyway, so I think they deserve to know as soon as you can realistically tell them. They'll want to know and they will often be able to offer help and support that you need.

For your employer, I'd say 'the sooner the better'. What is to be gained by keeping employers waiting before they can plan, or family and friends wondering what is wrong and possibly imagining even worse things than those that are going on?

As soon as you know the diagnosis, treatment plan and a rough timetable for treatment, I think it helps to share this, in confidence, with your employer.

Friends can be told in stages, depending on how close you are, how relevant it is for them to know early on and also in terms of the help and support they can offer you at this time. Modern equipment makes a circular letter easy to produce and e-mail messages are perfectly acceptable to most people if you have this facility. Some will need a more personal approach. This takes more time and energy, so I simply apologised for any delay, explaining that I had not the energy to write too many letters in one day. Nobody minded. Everyone appreciated the smallest effort on my part to keep them informed.

This is also the time to look at your insurance policies. Some will state the period of time that must elapse before you can claim, during which time you probably receive your full salary from your employer. Other policies will pay immediately. Check them now and make a note of the earliest dates that you can submit your claims.

How do I tell them?

I cannot claim to be a lover of history, but I believe that during battles at sea it was common to fire a 'warning shot' across the ship before attacking the hull directly.

The same approach is helpful in this situation. Receiving a blunt e-mail message saying, '*Hi John, have cancer. Regards. Mary*' on a Monday morning is probably not the best way for John to start his working week!

There are various ways of sharing the news. One could say things like this, building the story over a few days:

- 'I am having some tests and am a bit worried. I'll know more in a day or two.'
- 'I have been told that I will probably need quite a long period of treatment.'
- 'The doctor has told me that I definitely have cancer. We'll know more in a few days.'

And so one can share the news in a controlled manner, being honest but not giving all the information at once.

At other times the straightforward approach I adopted might be appropriate. It depends on your circumstances. I think the main thing is to be honest, open and accurate.

Telling children is a different matter and we looked at that in Chapter 31.

Where should they be told?

This sounds a strange question!

For the person hearing the bad news, the easiest way is in person, in a place familiar to both parties and not in a hurry. The hearer will be shocked, embarrassed, upset and unsure what to say. There will be silences. They may want to touch you to express their care and concern because they are lost for words.

For you, a letter allows you to choose your words carefully and to know that you said exactly what you wanted to and had the chance to compose the message carefully. Giving it verbally is not so easy and it will probably 'come out all wrong' – I know because I've been there!

I think the telephone is worst of all. You speak: there is a stunned silence. Do you continue? Do you ask if they heard what you said? What is their face saying that they can't express in words? It's not easy, but it may be unavoidable.

If there is any doubt that the verbal message was heard, especially when using the telephone, I suggest that you follow up that message with a letter. My late mother was rather deaf and I am sure it was when I wrote to my parents, confirming what I had told them, that the truth dawned fully. I am glad my brother was there to support them.

Note

There is so much going on that it is impossible to keep track of everything. I found that a notebook or pad of paper was very helpful for jotting things down and returning to them later on. In the initial days of my first illness almost ten years ago, I started keeping a diary. I basically recorded everything that might be relevant. I have been amazed at how useful it was.

It might help to sit and write some notes about any major plans you have for your family, holidays or work and also your plans and aspirations. You'll need your diary too.

Use a different page for each item you identify. Label the page and re-visit these topics later on when you are better able to plan ahead.

Keep records of when you visited the doctor and hospital. Insurance companies have a habit of asking for this information and I am thankful that I recorded these details.

Keep a record of any health or income protection insurance claims you make. If you don't use a word-processor or computer, obtain photocopies of any letters you send.

Speaking from personal experience, I suggest that you keep all these records together and keep them for a long time. They could be an important reminder of the information you had available at the time.

Do

When you have to tell a vulnerable person your bad news, it's good to be aware that they might need someone to turn to for support. Make sure that they know that it is OK with you for them to tell that person why they are upset and need comfort or support. If you don't give this 'permission', they might feel unable to talk and could become very isolated and find it even harder to cope.

If you anticipate problems, especially with aged parents or people who will have difficulty coping with news that they must hear, it might help if you can speak to one of their friends first to elicit their help in readiness for the stressful time ahead of your relative. I am sure the person won't mind: in fact I think they will be pleased to help.

If you care for someone who is dependent on you for practical help, which you will now be unable to give, do not just sit feeling guilty. Seek advice about the kinds of assistance that are available. It is not your fault and it is not something you chose to do. The GP practice or social worker may be able to advise you about suitable and appropriate services available and you will know that they will understand the needs of the person you care for and will address all the issues needing to be resolved.

Explore

There are several books available from public libraries and bookshops about coping with difficult times and sharing bad news with others. What suits one person is not the choice of another. I suggest that you browse in your local library before spending money on these resources.

More Information

Telling people bad news is exhausting and stressful. You may feel pressure to share the information with everyone as quickly as possible, but do remember that you are probably emotionally and physically exhausted and you need support too.

Prioritise the order in which people need to know your news and pace yourself. Allow time for yourself and accept the help that is offered to you.

If you are like me, you'll feel guilty for not being at work and for 'letting people down'!

People will react to your news in different ways. Some will be very supportive while others who can't cope with it will possibly keep a distance because they hurt for you and just don't know what to say.

Chapter 33

I am 'hurting' because of my illness

The doctor says

When we think of hurting or pain, we usually think of the physical sensation but there are other ways in which we 'hurt'.

Dame Cicely Saunders, founder of St Christopher's Hospice and pioneer in the development of hospices in Britain, taught about four types of suffering that make up one's 'total pain' or 'total suffering'. These four are:

- physical pain – which we have briefly looked at
- social pain
- emotional pain
- spiritual pain.

Social pain

What do we mean by 'social pain'? Well, it's a way of acknowledging how your illness affects your day-to-day life. Having to look through your diary and cancel plans or write a letter to friends telling them you are ill is *'social pain'*.

The effect your illness has on your family is also an example of social pain.

Emotional pain

Think back to the day when you were first told that you had cancer. Did you think 'Why me?' or something similar? Being given bad news hurts – it might not hurt physically, but it hurts psychologically and emotionally.

Spiritual pain

In the medical sense, 'spirituality' is more than just religion. Spirituality is often defined as 'that which has a meaning'.

Looking at my own past, having an active personal Christian faith has helped me through both my experiences of cancer. My whole career changed the first time I had cancer. At the time I wondered what was going on but, looking back, I believe God had a plan for my life. I have no regrets about having had cancer. Because our children were still quite young, my wife was not working during my first illness. The two years I was off work are among the best we have had in the 27 years since we met.

As for the present, I don't know why I have had to be treated for cancer for a third time, but it meant that I had time to do things I otherwise would not have done. Writing this book has been in my mind for years. If you are reading this, that means that my work did get published and it was that second illness that afforded me the opportunity to start and my third illness that saw the work completed.

Yes, I did ask God what He was doing. I learned that He does not always answer such questions, but I believe that my faith is stronger as a result of my cancer. Illness can be an enriching experience – not always at the time, but afterwards.

Think

Social pain

☐	Are you able to work?
☐	Have you lost your usual role in the family – are you the 'breadwinner'?
☐	Can you get out and meet friends or go out socially?

Not being able to do these things hurts!

Emotional pain

There are lots of 'emotional pains' along the journey and if these are not resolved they can make your physical pain feel worse.

Being sad or feeling depressed (*see* Chapter 11) makes our physical pain seem more severe.

☐	Are you feeling sad or depressed?

Spiritual pain

Spiritual pain is sometimes thought of in three parts – past, present and future.

☐	Thinking of the past, are there things that you regret or feel guilty about?
☐	How are you coping with the present? Do you feel isolated or are you struggling to cope? Does this illness feel unfair and make you angry; with yourself for not coping, with someone else who possibly put you at risk of developing the disease, or simply angry with God?
☐	How do you see your future? Does it fill you with fear? Does it all seem hopeless and pointless?

I once heard a hospital chaplain ask a patient, 'What is the source of your spiritual comfort? Is it:

- certain, present and real now?
- uncertain?
- lost temporarily or permanently?'

This is all part of the 'total pain' you are feeling just now.

Physical pain

Having to deal with the social, emotional and spiritual effects of our illness causes us anxiety and stress, which in turn may make our physical pain feel more severe by reducing our ability to cope with it. We looked at this in Chapter 1 'How can my pain be assessed?'

Ask

Look at the 'Think' section again. Have you ticked any of the boxes, indicating that you might be suffering socially, emotionally or spiritually? If so, ask for help from family, friends, a social worker, counsellor, minister or other religious adviser as appropriate.

If you think your perception or tolerance of physical pain may be affected by any of these, you could be right. This is another reason to seek appropriate advice for these aspects of your 'total suffering'.

Note

Make a note of any questions you need to ask or issues you need to resolve. Note any names or telephone numbers in order to obtain the help you need.

Do

My message here is not so much a checklist of things to do but simply to encourage you to deal with these issues now. They affect your quality of life and are just as important as any other issue you are currently facing.

Explore

The main thing to explore is how to find the peace of mind you seek. For me it comes from my faith in God.

More Information

The concept of 'total suffering' is not widely explored beyond textbooks on hospice and palliative care, but it really fits all aspects of our lives. It affects your relatives too – they are suffering psychologically, socially and spiritually as a result of your illness.

Chapter 34

I look different since my operation

The doctor says

Our son, Chris, was 2½ when his little sister Sharon was born. When the doctor (Martin, my senior partner in the practice) came to check that Alice was well, he bent over the cot to look at Sharon. Chris stood watching in fascination, and then he spoke. 'Uncle Martin,' he said, examining Martin's bald head, 'did you cry when your hair fell out?'

We stood in silence, unsure what to say. Martin laughed and, taking Chris on his knee, replied, 'I can't remember, it fell out a long time ago.'

A few years later, I did not cry when all my hair fell out after chemotherapy, but I did feel very aware of how my appearance had suddenly changed. It made me think of the famous statement made by Jean Cocteau, who said that, '*Mirrors should think for longer before they reflect.*'

Think

Perhaps you can relate to Jean Cocteau's comment. People will probably be fully aware of your changed appearance, even if they make no comment. How should you deal with this?

If your appearance has changed in a way that is reasonably obvious, such as hair loss, for which you now wear a wig, there are two possible ways to cope with this:

- Acknowledge it and encourage open conversation about it.
- Ignore it and pretend that it is not happening.

I find that the former method breaks down barriers and allows openness, which is easier in the long term.

For less obvious loss of body parts, such as a breast, this loss will be obvious to you and your spouse or partner but, with modern garments, a stranger need not be aware of it. Whether you choose to let people know is up to you. It is all about how much to tell people, but do make sure that you keep a record of what you tell specific individuals if you really are concerned about protecting your privacy. You might wish to look at Chapter 32 'How do I tell others the bad news?'

It is easy to think that it is mainly women who have to face the issue of disfiguring surgery and loss of a body part. A few moments' reflection will remind us that this is not so. When I was attending hospital last week, I saw a man in a wheelchair who had just lost one of his legs below the knee. That is an obvious loss, but people are also affected by the less obvious losses. Let me share a true story.

I recall an ex-serviceman who had refused surgery for lung cancer. He told me that he could have coped with any wounds received in the defence of his country, but to see a scar on his chest, as a daily reminder of his cancer, would have been unbearable.

When I shared this with other men who had scars from operations, some admitted that they did not like to see the scar because either they did not like their altered appearance or it was a painful reminder of previous illness. Others accepted it better.

There is no 'right' way to cope with seeing an operation wound every day. It is a reminder of your illness. I know – I see my scars every day. Most days I accept them or ignore them but on some days I have negative feelings about them. Most of the time I am thankful that the scar is a reminder of a tumour that has been removed and therefore unable to do any more damage. Sometimes I am tempted to ask why it all happened. I don't get any answers.

Ask

You know how you feel about yourself, but do you really *know* what others think? If this matters to you, you probably need to ask them!

Ask your partner or spouse

This will not be easy for either of you, but, until you ask, you will not know your partner's true feelings. It takes time to adjust to your altered appearance, but together you can work coming to terms with these changes.

Many women can accept their loss of a breast and be thankful for the life-saving effect of the operation. Others feel cheated and less attractive. Some fear that they will experience difficulties in their marriages.

Most husbands I spoke to were so pleased that their wives were alive and well that they regarded their altered appearance as a secondary issue.

Similarly, men who felt less manly, owing for example to the loss of a testicle, were more worried than their partners in most cases. In most cases, the issue that is raised here is that of having children. Sperm collection and storage before surgery or chemotherapy is often possible.

Ask the doctor or nurse

Sometimes it is possible to have reconstructive surgery, for example after breast cancer treatment. This will not usually be done immediately and it may not be possible to fulfil all your expectations and hopes for a completely satisfactory reconstruction. You must ask for expert advice on this matter.

There are many specialist nurses available to advise you about all aspects of your altered appearance after surgery. Many techniques are available to help you restore an acceptable appearance and help you gain confidence to go out and to be in company again, e.g. after bowel surgery.

Ask patients and friends

You might find it helpful to speak to other patients who have had similar surgery. Some patients willingly make themselves available to other patients for this type of discussion. They have probably experienced the same emotions as you are going through and they might be able to share ideas and thoughts that will help you cope with the problems you are facing.

A trusted friend might be willing to be your confidant. Their support can be invaluable. They might not be able to fully understand how you are feeling but can offer support and friendship at a difficult time.

Ask specialist advisers

You might want to ask about suitable clothing after a mastectomy or bowel surgery requiring a bag. Many people who have had disfiguring surgery or who have to wear a colostomy bag after bowel surgery take up sporting activities again. Specially designed swimwear and sportswear is available to help you disguise any loss of body parts or help you start living a normal life again. See 'Explore' for more details of a few companies but do ask the nurse specialist who can advise you about other services suited to your needs.

Ask advice and support groups

Help is also available in the form of support networks for almost every kind of cancer resulting in a change in your appearance. There are too many to list here and the contact details can change, but organisations like CancerLine, a charity associated with Macmillan Cancer Relief, keep updated details for all the local support groups listed in the country. CancerLine can be contacted confidentially and free of charge during office hours by ringing 0800 808 2020.

Note

Make a note of any people, organisations or manufacturers that you think might be able to help you. Often this information is available at the clinic, sometimes it will be given to you and occasionally you'll see something in a magazine and may want to explore it later. Make a note of it now and come back to it when you want to and are ready to do so.

Do

You might lose interest in intimate relationships due to other problems including pain (*see* Chapters 1–5), tiredness (*see* Chapter 26), and feeling sick or vomiting (*see* Chapter 21). A wound that will not heal may also make you feel unacceptable to your partner (*see* Chapter 29).

After chemotherapy or radiotherapy, exhaustion and loss of libido are not uncommon, but these usually recover after a while. A swollen abdomen (*see* Chapter 25) might cause physical problems as well as altering your normal appearance.

Even if you feel unattractive, you still need to be loved and cared for. Even if you are too tired for full intercourse, couples can express their love by being cuddled and held close in a loving embrace. As time progresses, you may feel stronger, but the important thing is to express your love for each other and to appreciate that true beauty is more than skin deep.

Explore ways of expressing your emotions, your love and your care for those whom you love.

For many couples, closeness is especially important in times of illness. Feeling loved, valued and special to the person you love has several positive effects. Such closeness:

- allows a feeling of normality, of being loved, in spite of a changed appearance
- gives a feeling of security and warmth and being valued
- improves self-esteem and emotional stability
- can make pain seem less intense.

Explore

Various magazines and papers will carry advertisements for mastectomy bras, etc. Many people have been satisfied with their products. There are also companies, recognised by the specialist teams, which offer personalised fittings.

A couple of suppliers are listed here, with their specialist services annotated. There are many others, but space would not allow me to include them all. As with everything else, people retire and go out of business, but I did check that these firms were all active at the time of going to press. If they are not trading now, ask the appropriate specialist nurse for up-to-date advice.

Breast surgery

Eloise Lingerie, PO Box 70, Bury St Edmunds, Suffolk IP30 0JT. Tel. 01284 828787.

One-to-one telephone advice, personal fittings by appointment and a free catalogue are among the services offered.

Colostomy or ileostomy

Specially designed sportswear and swimwear is available for people with a colostomy or ileostomy bag following surgery. Contact Geoffrey Vaughan (tel. 01827 66854) for further details.

More Information

The artist John Constable (1776–1837) said, 'There is nothing ugly; I never saw an ugly thing in my life for, let the form of an object be what it may, light, shade and perspective will always make it beautiful.'

The old proverb says, 'The peacock has fair feathers but foul feet.' When did you last study a peacock's feet? We generally admire the wonderful tail feathers. If you do feel inclined to study the peacock's feet, while they are not as attractive as its tail, they have many fascinating design features perfectly suited to the bird's natural habitat.

The last peacock I looked at had, on closer inspection, several damaged tail feathers. This did not take away from his overall beauty. His confidence to join us and share our picnic lunch endeared him to us. There's a lot more to a peacock than his tail. Allow yourself to see the 'whole you' and encourage others to do likewise.

Chapter 35

I would like to return to work

The doctor says

One of the things I craved was 'normality'. I know other patients have expressed the same wish – to get back to work, be able to drive, work in the garden, finish that DIY project and so on.

Returning to work means that we are getting better, regaining control and that things are 'looking up'. In my case, because my immune system was suppressed and I was at risk of picking up a life-threatening infection, I never returned to my original job, but was very fortunate in being offered a post in medical education, specialising in cancer and palliative care.

So, even if you can't return to your normal job, there may be other options.

Think

Think about your general fitness, energy levels and stamina. How physically demanding is your job?

- Are you considering resuming work full-time or part-time?
- Are you able to be active all day at present without needing to rest?
- How is your concentration for work, driving, etc?
- If you did resume work and were unable to cope, what options are open to you?
- Are there any rehabilitation schemes available and suitable for you?

Ask

Going back to work after a period of absence and treatment for a serious illness is big decision. You might like to find out about the following issues.

- Can you begin with part-time work and increase as you build up your stamina?
- What happens if you can't cope and go off sick again?
- If you are approaching retirement age, is there the option of an early retirement on the grounds of your health? How would this affect your pension?
- What rehabilitation and re-training is available to you?
- If you have a private permanent health insurance or similar cover, what happens if you resume work and cannot cope? Is there a qualifying period before you can claim again?

Note

Make a note of any issues that you need to discuss with your employer, insurance companies, your accountant or the tax office. Make a note of any advice they give you as there may be issues that you are not aware of. The law seems to change frequently and it is hard to keep up-to-date.

Do

Investigate fully all the options open to you concerning part-time work, full-time work and early retirement. Think about your diagnosis and whether there is any significant risk of the cancer recurring.

Keep clear and accurate records of all discussions and try and obtain everything in writing. My experience is that telephone advice can be misunderstood. I certainly seemed to misunderstand the 'rules' I thought I was told over the phone! The regulations for payment of benefit may change, as may your individual circumstances, so keep accurate notes in case anything is questioned later. My Inland Revenue accounts took almost two years to finalise and had I not kept good notes I would have had great difficulty remembering what was going on at the time.

Explore

Before deciding to resume work, look carefully at the alternatives. Could you retire? Is it possible to pay off the mortgage and enjoy some free time or take up a part-time job that you would enjoy and that would provide enough money to live comfortably but without the stress of your former employment?

If resuming work means having to move house or invest in expensive new equipment, there may be unforeseen difficulties in making these changes. Explore all the aspects before making a final decision.

If you must change jobs, find out about availability of funds for re-training or setting up a new business.

More Information

After being given a diagnosis of cancer, you will probably have great difficulty in obtaining a new life insurance policy or applying for a new mortgage. It is very unusual for a patient who has been treated for cancer to be offered 'standard' premiums and you may find that you are refused life insurance cover for a mortgage. There are, however, specialist companies that offer 'high risk' insurance cover – but it is likely to be quite expensive.

Even payment protection for a credit agreement may be refused on the grounds of your past medical history if the credit card company considers it likely that you will be unable to meet the payments due to a recurrence of your illness.

Chapter 36

I don't think my illness is as serious as they say

The doctor says

None of us wants to be given bad news. Being given bad news is very different from reading a newspaper headline; it is personal. We can't walk away from it. It is my bad news, your bad news, and while we do not want to accept it, we must. We must also come to terms with the fact that, however much we dislike what we heard, it will not go away.

One of the basic ways in which we sometimes cope is to convince ourselves that something is not happening to us. This is called 'denial'. In the short term, denial allows us time to come to terms with what is happening.

Denial is a primitive defence mechanism which we use to cope when we have to face very distressing events or thoughts. This helps us adjust to the event and become accustomed to a major loss before responding to the painful reality of the situation, e.g. accepting the fact that we have cancer.

Don't think I am blaming anyone who copes in this way. The very first day I went to hospital to see the consultant, when he said that he would see me in his ward three hours later, I told him that I was on my way to see two patients at home.

In response he said, 'You are playing for time, using denial as a means of trying to find some way round this. You need that operation tomorrow at 9 a.m. Go home and pack your bags and let someone else do the work – you'll not be there for a while!'

What he said was perfectly true. I would rather have been anywhere else at that time and I did not want to face the fact that I knew deep down I had cancer.

Who does want to face such news?

Think

If you think your illness is less serious than you have been told, think about these questions.

- Who told you the diagnosis?
- Had they the results of all the tests and investigations you have had?
- Thinking about the symptoms that made you attend the doctor, were you given any other possible cause for these? Has that possibility been completely ruled out?
- If you attended a screening clinic and your diagnosis was made after this, are you worried that there might be a mistake because you feel too well and had no reason to think you were suffering from any illness? (This is the value of

screening clinics; diseases are detected at a very early stage, often before you feel unwell.)

- Do you just find it all too hard to believe and take in?
- Do you feel threatened by the thought of the illness and the treatment and just want it all to be a mistake?

Ask

If there are questions burning in your mind, you really need to ask for advice and help. Do you need to ask any of the following questions, or others that you have thought of that are not listed here?

- Is the diagnosis right: could there be any mistake?
- Is it really cancer? Could it be something else – a less serious problem?
- Can I feel so well and really have cancer?
- Would more tests help?
- Would someone else tell me something different?

All the necessary tests will have been done. Some tests are very invasive and uncomfortable and some involve exposure to x-rays. The doctors will not repeat tests that expose you to such discomfort or unnecessary radiation without a very good reason.

Asking for a second opinion in the hope of being told something else is, quite simply, a waste of time and resources. I have never seen a diagnosis changed as a result and any delay in starting treatment could put you at serious risk.

Note

Make a note of anything you have been told, who said it, and on what basis. When you look at these notes later, you will be able to make a better judgement about the accuracy of what you were told. It is likely that you will be able to relate the information given to the results of tests carried out. In the very unlikely event that there is a difference in the message you are given, you will be able to trace back to find where, when and why the misunderstanding arose.

Do

Allow others to help. Being told that you have a serious illness and attending hospital for tests and treatments is very stressful and wearing.

Take your medication exactly as prescribed, even if you are awaiting confirmation of your diagnosis. Attend all clinic appointments and resist the temptation to go to another practitioner for a second opinion. The chances of the diagnosis being wrong are very small and delays in treatment can be costly to you.

Accept support and help – social, practical and psychological. You are not weak or feeble for accepting help. You are human.

Explore

You will probably be tempted to explore all the possible diagnoses and treatment options. My experience is that doing this is unhelpful. With, literally, millions of web sites dealing with cancer, where does one start? I am not aware of any way of obtaining a personal, accurate diagnosis and treatment plan except by seeing a doctor and trusting them to do what is best and right for you. It is very easy to find inaccurate or irrelevant information.

More Information

Doctors sometimes break our use of denial as a coping mechanism into two types – 'healthy denial' and 'unhealthy denial'. What do they mean by these terms?

Healthy denial allows patients to manage the unwanted situations that we cannot change and gives us time to become accustomed to our new problems before responding to the major changes that are associated with our new situation.

Overall, we are moving on, coping most of the time, accepting what is happening and getting on with our treatment, even though we may hate what we have to go through.

Unhealthy denial is when the way we react acts as a barrier and we simply can't adjust to our new situation. We say 'it just can't be true' and 'it can't be happening to me'. We may be unaware of it but our family, the doctor and nurse will recognise that we are not coping with the illness and are at risk. If it is not dealt with, the situation can become bad enough to endanger our personal best interests or our treatment.

In such cases, the doctors and nurses may wish to talk with you if they recognise that you are having difficulty accepting what is happening to you. In this event, they will probably:

- explore the issues you would rather not have to think about
- invite you to discuss your thoughts and anxieties
- ask whether you feel depressed or anxious because of pain or other symptoms
- ask for your permission to talk with your relatives and advise them about how to help and support you at this very stressful time.

Do not feel guilty about this. It's a perfectly normal, but slightly unusual, way for our bodies to react to a very threatening situation. You are not going mad!

Chapter 37

I don't want to talk to the doctor or nurse any more

The doctor says

When patients stop talking to the staff, it is natural for the staff to wonder why. Staff will be asking themselves if they have hurt your feelings or upset you in some way. They might need to explore these possibilities and, in so doing, are not trying to force you to talk or enter into discussion against your wishes. They simply need to know that they are not responsible for something that they need to resolve.

Think

Why do you not want to talk any more?

☐ Are you confused or do you feel that you are being given conflicting information by different people and see no point in asking questions or talking?

☐ Are you feeling depressed and do not wish to talk (*see* Chapter 11)?

☐ Are you feeling too tired to be bothered talking (*see* Chapter 26)?

☐ Has your pain become worse (*see* Chapters 1–5)?

☐ Is there some other symptom bothering you, but you are embarrassed to talk about it?

☐ Do you think that your problems are not as serious as someone else's and you should not engage busy staff in conversation about your problems?

☐ Did something happen that makes it difficult for you to talk to the staff now?

☐ Did you disclose something last time that you now wish you had not said?

☐ Do you have a better rapport with some members of staff than others?

Ask

If you have been given information that seems to be contradictory, you must ask for clarification. It is almost always a simple misunderstanding or difference in use of words or terminology, but while it festers in your mind you suffer an added stress.

If pain, increasing tiredness, depression, or some other physical problem is bothering you, ask for help. These can almost always be treated and your quality of life improved. Not reporting a problem simply means it doesn't get dealt with. You are not a 'nuisance' for reporting that you need help. That's what the staff are trained to do and it's why they are there.

If you are upset or embarrassed about something you said, try and see the appropriate person and 'clear the air'. It's seldom as bad as it seems and nobody will expect you to be able always to say the right thing, in the right way, when you are under the stress you are facing just now.

If you disclosed something you'd rather have kept to yourself, staff will respect your confidentiality and you need only to ask that it is not recorded or shared.

Note

There is not a lot to note here, except perhaps any conflicting information that might need clarification.

Do

Try and recognise that when patients stop talking the staff may be wondering why and asking themselves whether they have been responsible for causing some offence.

It may be necessary for you to explain that you simply do not feel like talking. The staff will probably feel some need to check the reason for this – things that are included in the 'Think' list above. This is their job – they are not being 'nosy'.

If you feel that there is some kind of barrier or difficulty between an individual staff member and yourself, this can be difficult to overcome. Personality differences will always exist, but don't let that be a reason for you to suffer simply by refusing to report any problems to this individual.

Let your family know that you are not feeling like conversation and in-depth discussion. It helps if you can let them know why you feel this way.

If appropriate, nominate a suitable person to answer phone calls for you and allow you to enjoy peace and quiet if you don't want to talk to visitors for a while.

Explore

Do you need to talk but are not sure who you need to talk to? Are there issues that you need to discuss but you 'don't know where to start'?

- Counsellors can help you if you are having problems coping with your illness.
- Ministers are very happy to come and discuss any religious or spiritual issues (*see* Chapter 43).
- Social workers can help with financial issues.
- Solicitors readily visit homes, hospitals or hospices to help with making a will (*see* Chapter 44).
- Specialist nurses, e.g. Macmillan nurses and Marie Curie nurses, are available to discuss practical care and other specialist help.

These are but a few of the people who can help. If you feel you need to talk to one or more of these people, ask the nurse or doctor who is available to help you.

More Information

Staff depend very much on the conversation that goes on between patients and themselves to know how you are feeling, how well treatment is working and generally how to provide the best service to you. When a patient refuses to talk or discontinues a conversation the staff can feel lost and quite powerless to help.

Your decision to be quiet may be having more widespread effects than you realise!

Chapter 38

I would like to try complementary (alternative) therapy

The doctor says

People often assume that, because I am a doctor, I would never even think of using complementary (alternative) medicines or therapies. They are wrong! I have used complementary therapies for myself and even prescribed them for others. Having said this, I have not undertaken the full training course in any of the complementary therapies, but have attended some short courses so that I had a 'working knowledge'.

When I was a medical student, there was 'orthodox medicine' (which I was studying) and 'alternative medicine', which I viewed with some suspicion! I never heard it referred to as 'complementary therapy' until some time later.

I was on a short training course on homoeopathic medicine once and noticed the word 'TEETH' written on the letter from the patient's GP. Since there was no mention of any dental problem, I asked what the reference to teeth was about.

The consultant replied, 'It's my shorthand for "Tried Everything Else, Try Homoeopathy!"' She went on to explain that this was how many patients and some doctors saw the role of homoeopathy – a last resort.

The older term 'alternative medicine' implied that you had a choice of 'either this or that'. The modern name 'complementary therapy' is better because it reminds us that you can sometimes use traditional medicines and treatments in combination with complementary therapy. I say sometimes, because many of the agents used in complementary therapy are very powerful and can interfere with prescribed medications.

I am aware that advice on complementary therapy can be obtained from a variety of sources – shops, magazines and the Internet, to name but three. I once decided to seek advice about a particular complementary therapy. I went along, explained my problem and was slightly taken aback when the person advising me showed absolutely no knowledge of the cause of my problem but offered a menu of possible 'cures' from which I was invited to 'make my own choice'. My choice was to make my exit!

I was trained to find the cause of the problem and choose treatment that deals specifically with that cause.

The moral of the story is, make sure the practitioner you consult is properly qualified and registered. The appropriate professional bodies that can advise you about this are listed in the 'Useful organisations' section at the back of the book.

Think

Why are you considering using complementary therapy?

☐ Is it to help you relax and maximise your quality of life?
☐ Are you thinking of stopping a clearly beneficial conventional treatment? Why?
☐ Is there any reason why complementary therapy is not advisable for you? If in any doubt, ask!

☐ Have you made enquiries about the cost of the treatment?
☐ Are there any reported risks or side effects associated with the complementary therapy you are considering? Is it of any *proven* value?
☐ Is written information on complementary therapies, from reputable sources, available to you?
☐ Does your doctor or the hospital have access to a complementary therapist, or have you obtained the names of local certified practitioners?

Ask

- Find out how your doctors and nurses involved in your care view the complementary treatments on offer. Is there any risk of an interaction between the orthodox and complementary treatments? (This information can be difficult for doctors to find and is not routinely sent to them.)
- Check that using a complementary treatment need not delay or stop the use of conventional therapies.
- Ask the doctor or nurse if they know of a certified practitioner in your area.
- Check that you can see your usual doctor afterwards to report whether it was helpful.

Note

Complementary therapies often involve dealing with the physical, social, psychological and spiritual aspects of your self and your illness.

There will be many questions asked that you might not have thought of before. Make a note of anything that you need to explore further. Think about which of the four aspects of your problem this addresses and decide who can help you most. *See* Chapter 33 'I am "hurting" because of my illness'.

Do

Continue to take your prescribed medicines exactly as you were told to do by the doctor or nurse. If a complementary practitioner advises you to alter the way in which you take your prescribed medicines, do not make any changes until you have consulted your doctor. Most complementary therapists are not medically qualified, so you are quite justified in questioning their judgement if they tell you to discontinue or amend the medication prescribed by your GP or hospital doctor.

Make sure you tell both the doctor and the complementary therapy practitioner about all aspects of your illness and treatment. Mistakes can be made if any information is withheld and there will be only one person blamed for that – you!

Explore

Before embarking on any course of complementary treatment, check that the practitioner is registered with and approved by the appropriate professional body. There are unqualified persons making claims about their expertise, which are unfounded, so check first. The 'Useful organisations' section at the back gives details of a selection of statutory bodies to help you.

The UK Nursing and Midwifery Council issued new guidelines on the use of complementary therapy in June 2003. These relate to safety and ensuring that therapists are appropriately trained.

There is a wealth of information in the books in local libraries. There is also a great demand for complementary therapies which has resulted in many ineffective remedies being sold over the counter. Check what you are being offered and avoid wasting your money on an unproven, untested product.

More Information

There is a diverse assortment of complementary therapies, from the ancient (e.g. acupuncture) to the modern (biofeedback). Some offer fundamental curative treatment (naturopathy), while others place more emphasis on symptomatic remedies (homoeopathy). Some reject all forms of 'artificial' help as unnecessary (nature cure) while others use extensive medicinal intervention (e.g. herbalism).

On the subject of herbal remedies, a single herb could contain hundreds of different chemicals about which little is known. It is almost impossible to identify all the chemical ingredients, many of which could be incompatible with your prescribed medications. They are best avoided.

Chapter 39

Why is my treatment not working?

The doctor says

Having to think about this question is very distressing. Having to ask it is even worse.

I have never had to ask this myself as a patient, but I have had to answer it.

There are several things one needs to consider. Among these are the questions:

- What was the treatment actually meant to achieve?
- Was the intended outcome a cure, or was it to relieve symptoms?

It is very easy to think that being offered treatment automatically means that there is hope of a cure. That is what we all want. Sadly it is not always possible.

Sometimes the cancer simply does not respond to the treatment. The doctors do not always know whether it will respond or not. There may have been more than one treatment to choose from and the one thought best for you will have been chosen. Cancer is a disease that doesn't always behave as one expects and, for that reason, the treatment seen as the best choice for you may actually not live up to expectations. There might be other options but, sadly, this is not always so.

Sometimes the only option is to try and relieve your symptoms and improve your quality of life.

Think

- Why do you think your treatment is not working? Do you feel less well or are you aware of a lump or bump that has started to grow or enlarge recently? Think about all the things that are making you suspicious that the treatment is not working.
- What were you told about the treatment you have been having? Was it intended to be a cure, or was it to relieve your symptoms? This discussion may have taken place some time ago. We all know how difficult it is to remember what was said and your circumstances may have changed since then. Try and recall all the relevant conversations. If you had someone with you, ask them too.
- When were you told about the treatment that apparently is not working now? This is where you need your diary! If you simply can't remember, don't worry. The hospital will have all the details in your notes. The doctor will be able to tell you the relevant dates.
- Who gave you this information? Once again, this can be very difficult to remember. It's one reason why I keep a diary! It is important to think about this. You want to be sure that the information was given to you personally by a doctor looking after you and was not a general comment obtained from a web

site or from an information service. The advice may be good, but cannot be specific to you.

It is always easiest to remember the 'positive' things we hear. None of us wants to think about the less hopeful messages we might be given. This is something that the doctors will need to explore in some detail to confirm that you have correctly understood the information they gave you, as we discovered in the section on being given bad news.

Ask

It can be difficult to ask questions in this situation. Sometimes we don't really want to hear the answers. Here are some things you might choose to ask about.

- Was your treatment intended to be a cure, or was it intended to relieve symptoms?
- Is your treatment really not working? Why not?
- Is your disease progressing and there is no treatment that will *cure* you now?
- What happens now?

Note

In the two sections above, there are many things that you might wish to make notes about. Start compiling a list of questions and the various points you need to clarify.

Do

The things to do here are all included in the other sections – find out what you need to know, make notes and explore where you are going in your illness.

Explore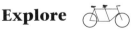

Be wary of all claims about 'miracle cures'. It takes, on average, 14 years for a new medicine to go from a new laboratory discovery to a licensed drug in the UK. Some other countries rush their new medicines through much faster than this and allow people to buy and try untested treatments much earlier. My personal belief is that this exposes the person to unacceptable risk.

You might wish to explore the options for your ongoing care and the support available for yourself and your family. I suggest that you do this through your GP and the hospital specialists.

More Information 📖

When you raise your concerns with the doctor, there are several things they will want to explore with you. These will probably include:

- establishing what you thought your treatment would achieve
- your understanding of the possible progression of your illness and its likely outcome.

It is quite likely that the doctor will need talk to you about:

- your understanding of what is happening with your cancer now
- your treatment to date and the options for your future treatment
- what other services and sources of help are available to you
- your thoughts about the future and the treatment options available.

Chapter 40

I feel like giving up

The doctor says

I have to confess to a certain fondness for Eeyore, that lovable but permanently depressed donkey created by AA Milne.

In one televised story, a very excited Piglet and Tigger are waiting by Eeyore's house when he wakens. They comment, 'Oh, Eeyore, you're awake.'

Eeyore replies, 'It happens every morning. I don't see why everyone's so excited about it!'

If you feel that your treatment is not working, you are tired and each treatment session seems to cause more side effects, it is understandable that you might feel a bit like Eeyore. Perhaps you feel like giving up.

Sometimes the treatment can leave you feeling far worse than you did when you first saw the doctor. This may make you feel like giving up, but do you really want to do so? If this phase is going to last for a few weeks, with improvement to follow, you probably can cope with it. You might be trying to take on too much at once and need just to take one day at a time. As the days pass and the treatment sessions come to an end, you may gradually feel better. That's what happened to me.

I must be realistic about the fact that there will come a time for some of us when we must recognise that treatment is not achieving the hoped-for outcome and our desire to give up is founded on the knowledge that we will not get better.

I said 'some of us' because, more and more, with successful treatments, people are dying with their cancer, not as a result of it. Older men with prostate cancer are a good example of this. So don't give up as soon as you are given your diagnosis!

Think

☐	How do you normally like to be treated when you are unwell? Do you like to be left alone or do you love to be fussed over?
☐	Do you accept that illness can make you unwell for a spell but that you will feel better soon, or do you feel depressed and find every illness very threatening?
☐	Are you having chemotherapy or radiotherapy at present? You might be feeling very tired and unwell because of these treatments.
☐	Is there something else happening that you are finding difficult? For example, are you in pain (see Chapters 1–5)?
☐	Are any other symptoms getting worse and are you afraid that they are going 'out of control'?
☐	Are you feeling depressed or sad (see Chapter 11)?

> ☐ Is your ongoing illness and treatment becoming too distressing?
> ☐ Do you feel 'out of control', with little or no choice in how your treatment and management plan is being decided? Do you wish to be more involved?
> ☐ Are you fully aware of your present condition and progress? Are you worried that you are not going to get better or do you think your treatment is not working (*see* Chapter 39)?

Ask

If you are you having chemotherapy or radiotherapy, ask if these may be responsible for how are feeling just now.

If you are in pain report it. Pain may become worse for a spell for various reasons and then improve again. Don't suffer in silence.

If you are afraid that some other symptom is going 'out of control', ask about it. Symptoms can seem worse when we are tired and feeling generally unwell due to chemotherapy and radiotherapy. Associated with this is the exhausting routine of attending hospital regularly.

Are you feeling depressed or sad? Speak to the nurse or doctor. Cancer treatment can make you feel quite low in spirits and 'down'.

Are you worried because you think you are not going to get better, or do you think your treatment is not working? Don't be afraid to ask when you will feel some benefit from the treatment and what it is meant to do.

If there is something else that you are finding difficult to cope with, ask about it.

Note

Make a note of any questions you want to ask. It can be hard to find the right words at the time, so it might help to write the question down now and be sure that you find out exactly what you need to know.

On the other hand, asking these kinds of questions might result in hearing things that you did not really want to be told.

Do

Concentrate on the things that you need to do. You have not got the energy to do everything, so accept help with tasks that you find difficult. I found it hard to admit that I was struggling to keep going but accepting help allowed me to focus on the most important things.

Make a list of the things you must do, and a list of things you would like to do. For each of these lists try and put a priority code next to each item. Tackle the important things, a little bit at a time. Allow yourself to be proud of what you have achieved.

Perhaps some things can be delegated and you can stop worrying about them.

Accept any practical or psychological support that may be appropriate. Perhaps you need to talk to someone who is not personally involved. If you think this might help, ask about seeing a counsellor. Do you think it might help to speak to your minister?

Explore

Find out if you are feeling unwell due to your present treatment. It may not be possible to change anything, but at least you'll have some idea of when you should start to feel better.

If the way you are feeling now is because your disease is progressing, there is almost certainly something that can be done to improve your quality of life. Do discuss your symptoms and problems with the doctor.

More Information

Modern healthcare recognises your rights as a patient. You have the right to discuss your treatment and how you wish to be looked after. If you wish to refuse treatment and 'give up', you have the right to do so, but this can put you at serious risk if continuing the treatment might have achieved a good outcome.

Before making any major decisions about whether or not to continue or give up, make sure you have discussed your feelings, the treatment options and all other relevant issues with your family and the doctor in charge of your care.

Chapter 41

I'm going into the hospice

The doctor says

Many people are unaware of the range of services offered in hospices today. Modern hospices offer day-patient units, specialist services, various clinics and in-patient beds for patients who require admission for control of symptoms, respite to allow their family a break or, in some cases, care at the end of life.

Too many people think that the last of these services is the only one offered.

The hospice staff specialise in managing the kinds of problems associated with cancer.

Contrary to what one might think, a lot of research goes on into finding better ways of managing symptoms experienced by cancer patients and the demand for education and teaching in this speciality is increasing.

Think

- What do you know about your local hospice and the services it provides?
- What do your relatives know about your local hospice and the services it provides?
- Why are you going into the hospice? Is it for:
  - respite care while your family has a short break?
  - assessment to see what services would be most appropriate for you?
  - expert assessment and management of a difficult symptom?
  - continuing care?

Ask

You might want to enquire about what services the hospice offers. They might offer:

- day care, with a range of services – bathing, specialist clinics, aromatherapy, relaxation, physiotherapy and others
- specialist nurses who could visit you at home
- respite care
- advice and help with difficult symptoms
- complementary therapies (*see* Chapter 38).

Ask what your admission is for and how long you are likely to be an in-patient.

Ask if the hospice has a brochure or a video that you could borrow. If you are well enough, perhaps you could arrange to visit the hospice and see for yourself what is available. This is a good opportunity to meet some of the staff and the visit will help you to find out much more.

It is becoming increasingly common for hospitals to prohibit smoking in the wards and even in the grounds. You may wish to ask about the hospice policy on smoking if this is something that you have found difficult in the past.

Do not be afraid to voice any anxieties you may have about the idea of going into a hospice. Many patients were unaware of what to expect and feared that they would find it a very disturbing experience. Most were pleasantly surprised by the number of patients who were preparing to go back home.

Note

As you think of things you want to know about the hospice, make a note of them and bring the list with you when you visit.

After your first visit, you will probably have many questions you will want to ask. Make a note of them as they arise.

Do

Find out what your relatives know about your local hospice and the services it provides. Correct any wrong ideas and misconceptions.

Be prepared to try something new! Many patients have learned that they had skills in painting, pottery and all kinds of activities they had never had time to explore!

If you are offered day care or another service that will help you or your family, think seriously about it. You will benefit from the specialist input. Many hospices have volunteer drivers who will take you to and from the hospice.

If you are going in for respite care and are reasonably well, your family might feel a bit guilty about going away for a few days for a short break. Discuss this with them and, if necessary, give them your 'permission' to go away, or even to be allowed to have a day off and not to feel obliged to visit you every day. Mobile phones allow freedom but easy contact. One does not have to go very far away for a holiday and both you and your family can benefit.

Explore

You may wish to find out more about the services offered by the hospice. While you may not need very much in the form of medical care, there are other people – social workers, chaplains and various therapists – who can help and advise about a range of issues that you might have been wondering about and not knowing whom to ask about.

More Information

Hospices do not usually accept patients who simply phone and ask to be allowed to attend. It is usually necessary for your GP to refer you to the hospice and a member of the hospice staff to assess how they can best help you.

Going into the hospice for a short respite break does not imply that you or your family are unable to cope. I have always said to families that our staff worked their shifts, went home and had their regular days off. Family carers do not have 'off duty' times. That's why hospices offer respite admissions.

Modern hospices are mostly specialist palliative care units, specialising in symptom control for patients with cancer and other serious illnesses. For this reason, long-term care is not always available. Many nursing homes are registered for the care of the terminally ill and can offer longer-term care if patients cannot be looked after at home. Your GP will have details of suitable local nursing homes.

Hospices aim to provide the highest possible standards of medical, nursing, social and spiritual care, with support from trained staff for a patient's family during the illness and for some time after the loss of a loved one.

Chapter 42

Will I be able to return home?

The doctor says

This is one of those questions that is probably more often thought than actually asked. It is a question that demands a proper answer, not just a response like, 'Of course you will.' The question needs to be carefully considered by the doctor or nurse who knows your individual needs and how well your needs can be met at home.

Think

- Why are you currently an in-patient? Is it for assessment, respite, symptom control or treatment?
- How well were you managing at home before you were admitted to the hospital or hospice where you are now?
- What problems did you encounter before your admission? Have these been resolved – either as a result of your stay in the hospital or hospice or by some other method?
- Will your family need extra support and help when you do get home?
- Think about the problems you might face concerning:
  - your mobility – do you need to use stairs and, if so, can you manage these?
  - the ease of getting to and from the bathroom – is it on the same floor?
  - whether you can wash and dress without help – how much help do you need?
  - whether your family can look after you and, if not, if appropriate help is available.

In your mind, work through the activities of a 'normal' day. Make a note of any difficulties you think of.

Ask

Ask about how feasible it is for you to get home. It might be worth asking your family or main carers to be present at such a discussion. Remember, the doctors and nurses are not allowed to discuss your illness with a third person without your permission, so it is important that you give your consent to such discussions.

If you have identified specific activities or problems with, for example, getting up and down stairs to the bedroom or bathroom, ask about whether it might be possible to borrow a bed and a commode that can be positioned downstairs, if this would allow you to return home.

Many problems can be overcome by the use of borrowed equipment, but you need to be aware that there are sometimes limited supplies of equipment and you might have to wait for someone else to return a borrowed item. For the same reason, it is essential that you promptly return anything you have on loan that you are no longer using. See 'Useful organisations' for some suppliers.

If it is agreed that you can go home, check what you should do if you cannot cope for any reason. Can your bed be kept for an agreed period – say 72 hours – in case you do not manage, so that you can be looked after by the same doctors and nurses? This is not always possible, so be very sure that you and those caring for you at home are happy with the decision.

Note

Look at the 'Think' section and make a note of any difficulties you anticipate when you return home. Discuss these with your family and the staff.

Make a note of any names and telephone numbers you are given for advice, help or borrowing equipment.

Make a note of any contact numbers and the names of staff you should speak to in the event that you need to be re-admitted within an agreed time frame.

Do

There is not much else for you to do at this point, but your family might need to think about moving beds or collecting equipment that you will need for your return home.

Make sure your family know exactly who is responsible for the supply of any equipment they can borrow and, if necessary, make a note of the relevant details to pass on to your relatives.

Explore

It's not very easy exploring practical issues from a hospital or hospice bed but you might be able to obtain some useful information from the social worker.

Your relatives or carers might wish to explore other possible resources for borrowing equipment. The Red Cross can also help with various items, but demand can exceed supply and there might be a waiting list. There's no harm in asking!

More Information

You need to be aware of what you are taking on in asking to go home. The doctor and nurse need to be very sure that you will be able to cope.

Before agreeing to let you return home, the doctor or nurse might need to discuss the question with the team who will be caring for you. They need to consider a number of things before giving you a final answer. These include:

- your fitness to cope at home
- whether your present condition is likely to change suddenly

- how well your family or carers will cope with your care – they don't work an eight-hour shift and then go home!
- availability of essential equipment
- availability of staff to help and support your family/carers – especially at weekends and public holidays.

It takes a few days to set up the arrangements for a community nurse to visit you at home and can take even longer for equipment to become available, be delivered and installed. This may be frustrating, but is less so than going home and failing to cope because everything was not ready for your return. That makes everyone lose confidence, which is the last thing you need. So, be patient!

Chapter 43

I want to think about my spiritual needs

The doctor says

It is increasingly recognised by the nursing and medical professions that the concept of 'spirituality' is not necessarily the same as being 'religious' and goes beyond religious affiliation, seeking a meaning and purpose in life, even among those who do not believe in God.

Your definition of spirituality may not include an allegiance to any formal religion. You may feel that your family and the people responsible for your care confuse what you see as 'spirituality' with 'religion'. You might need to clearly distinguish between your spiritual, religious and emotional needs.

In this chapter, we will think about both the meaning of your illness and the place of religious belief in your life.

Think

In his poem 'The Dry Salvages',[1] TS Eliot includes the line, 'We had the experience but missed the meaning.'

You have had the experience of illness. What is its meaning? Have you been searching for answers to the questions like 'Why me?', 'Why now?', and so on? If you are like me, you probably have not found any answers.

Are you seeking spiritual support? What exactly is it that you are asking for? Is it emotional support, help with searching for a meaning to your life and your present illness, or are you afraid to die without making peace with God?

I recognise that you may have no religious affiliation or you may belong to a different religion from the Christian faith, which is my own background. I can, however, only speak from a personal perspective.

For those nearing the end of life, there is commonly a spiritual need for forgiveness, reconciliation and affirmation of worth. You may be God-fearing or you may be fearing God. The Christian faith teaches that God sent His son Jesus to die a sacrificial death for our sins. The Bible says:

> For God so loved the world that He gave His one and only Son, that whoever believes in Him shall not perish but have eternal life.
>
> For God did not send His Son into the world to condemn the world, but to save the world through Him.
>
> Whoever believes in Him is not condemned, but whoever does not believe stands condemned already because he has not believed in the name of God's one and only Son.[2]

Therefore, those who genuinely seek God's forgiveness through Jesus' death for their sins will receive it and go to Heaven, but those who do not ask God's forgiveness are destined to eternal punishment.

Having accepted this forgiveness for myself many years ago, I believe that God controls my life and everything that happens to me. Of course, I ask questions, but I believe that God is in control and nothing will happen to me that He does not allow.

Ask

Having decided what type of help you actually are seeking, you need to ask the appropriate person to advise you.

If you are at home, it should be reasonably easy to find a minister or adviser from your particular faith and ask them to visit you.

The situation in hospitals is changing and there is an increasing tendency for the patient to have to 'make the first move' with respect to a visit from a chaplain. Don't wait for a chaplain to visit you automatically, speak to the nurses and ask them to arrange for you to be visited by the appropriate representative of your faith.

If you want a non-religious contact, ask the staff what arrangements they have for such a visit. Some hospitals have Spiritual Care Co-ordinators who visit and assess who is the best person to help with the broader issues of 'spirituality'.

Ask your family if they wish to be involved in any of these discussions. They are going through a stressful time and they might also find it helpful to meet with a spiritual adviser at this time.

Note

Make a note of any names and contact numbers you are given. You might not wish to pursue the matter just now, but it is always useful to have the details handy.

Do

In my experience, the relief and peace of mind experienced by patients who have spoken to someone about spiritual and religious issues has been obvious to family and staff alike.

On this basis, I would suggest that this is something that you should do sooner rather than later.

Explore

A World Health Organization Expert Committee on Palliative Care stated that patients have the right to expect that their spiritual experiences will be respected and listened to with attention.

It has been noted, in various studies over several years, that patients with a strong religious belief maintain their sense of control, hope and the meaning and purpose in life.[3]

You might wish to explore further the place of a personal faith in your life.

More Information

The World Health Organization points out that palliative care includes the control of pain, other symptoms, and psychosocial, social and spiritual problems.

The staff may not always share your views or beliefs, but they do not have to agree with people's beliefs or practices in order to take them seriously. Non-believers can affirm their contribution to a sense of wellbeing and integrity in others.

You should receive care that is non-sectarian, non-dogmatic and in keeping with your own views of the world.

References

1   Eliot TS (1963) The Dry Salvages. In: *Collected Poems 1909–1962*. Faber & Faber, London.
2   The Bible. *Gospel of John: Chapter 3, verses 16–18*. New International Version.
3   Koenig HG, Larson DB and Larson SS (2001) Religion and coping with serious medical illness. *Annals of Pharmacotherapeutics.* **35**(3): 352–9.

Chapter 44

I want to make a will

The doctor says

If you are like me, this is one of those tasks that is in a 'must do sometime' folder! It was my first cancer diagnosis that made Alice and me do something about a will and it gave us peace of mind having done it. It was much easier and cheaper than we expected.

Think

Why do you want to make a will now? Is it to:

- complete unfinished business?
- arrange disposal of your estate?

Both are very important.

If you are married and wish for your estate to be left to the spouse, it may not be strictly necessary to make a will, but dying intestate is more likely to give rise to problems for your spouse afterwards.

The situation regarding partners who are not married is more complex and is beyond the scope of this book.

Making a will may require two appointments with the solicitor. The first visit is for taking the instructions and the second is for signing the will. Fees depend on the amount of work and travelling involved.

Before speaking to a solicitor, spend some time thinking about all your assets. Is there an insurance policy that you have forgotten about?

Ask

- What advice is available regarding making a will?
- Is there a social worker who can give you advice, or is there any literature that will guide you through the basic process? The social worker cannot recommend an individual solicitor but can help you choose. They may be agreeable to contact a solicitor on your behalf if you are an in-patient and have difficulty making phone calls.
- Is there a family solicitor you could contact?
- Ask about what is involved in making the will.
- What personal papers do you need to have to hand?
- What is the approximate cost?
- Will the solicitor come to you if you are not fit to travel? Will this cost extra? The social worker might be able to advise you regarding the availability of voluntary solicitor services.

Note

Make a note of any insurance policies, pensions and other assets you have that might continue to be paid, or only become available for cashing in, after your death. Have you any bank accounts, bonds or other finances in accounts in your name only? If so, make notes of all the relevant details and discuss the best way to deal with these with the solicitor.

Do

In making a will, it is essential for an executor be appointed. He or she may be a beneficiary of the will. Two people, who cannot be beneficiaries, may need to witness your signature on your will.

Explore

Your will must be witnessed. If you have no family or close friends who can do this, ask if a member of staff can be your witness. Some hospitals do not allow medical and nursing staff to witness a patient's will. In this case, there is normally a nominated administrator who will assist. Find out about this before the solicitor visits to have the will signed and witnessed.

More Information

The doctor caring for you may be required to make a written statement that you are mentally competent to make a will, particularly if you are very unwell.

'Living wills' are dealt with in Chapter 45.

Chapter 45

Euthanasia, living wills (advance directives) and resuscitation

The doctor says

This is a complicated subject and one in which the law and public attitudes are changing. I have tried to reflect a variety of current opinions by quoting several points of view, mostly published in the few weeks before this book went to press. My own personal view is that euthanasia is morally wrong, and that, with good palliative care, one should not need to ask for an early death. I also am concerned that a premature death, at the hand of a third person and at a time of their choice, can deprive the patient of the opportunity of making peace with God before dying.

Here we will think about three issues – euthanasia, advance directives and instructions not to resuscitate.

Euthanasia

Euthanasia is an act intended to shorten life. It is classified as follows.

- Voluntary euthanasia is carried out at the specific request of a competent patient.
- Involuntary euthanasia is carried out without the request of a competent patient.
- Non-voluntary euthanasia is carried out when the patient is incapable of giving meaningful consent.

All forms of euthanasia are criminal acts in the UK.

Professor Tim Maughan[1] of the University of Wales College of Medicine points out that those in favour of euthanasia might argue on grounds of:

- compassion, saying that a death with dignity is preferable to suffering
- autonomy, arguing for the 'right to die'
- economics, because keeping people alive is expensive.

He also outlines the alternative viewpoint, namely that euthanasia is:

- unnecessary, because symptoms can usually be effectively controlled
- dangerous, because the terminally ill patient usually is vulnerable and may be poorly informed of the symptom control measures available
- regarded as morally wrong by most religious faiths and forbidden by all traditional codes of medical ethics.

Living wills (advance directives)

While a will is usually a document dealing with one's affairs regarding the funeral and the distribution of one's estate after death, you should be aware of the concept of the 'living will'.

Living wills, or 'advance directives', are the wishes of a person, recorded and witnessed at a time when they are in good health and of sound mind.

Living wills are frequently assumed only to instruct that no attempt should be made to prolong the patient's life in the event of illness such that they are deprived of quality of life and become a burden on others for their care.

Dr Michael Irwin,[2] a former Vice Chairman of the Voluntary Euthanasia Society, points out that an advance directive can equally state that a person wishes to be kept alive as long as possible and gives consent to all medical procedures necessary. A third type of living will may give consent only to measures directed at symptom control and freedom from pain.

Depending on its content, the document may have no legal status and may in fact request an action that is illegal in the UK.

This is an area where things are changing and if you are thinking of writing an advance directive you really must seek expert legal and medical advice. Don't forget that your family also should be aware of your wishes, but may not wish to carry them out.

'Do not resuscitate'

The instruction 'Do not resuscitate' may be considered acceptable in the event of a sudden collapse when it is thought likely that attempts to resuscitate will be unsuccessful or that you might only survive a very short time.

The British Medical Association and the Royal College of Nursing guidelines[3] on 'Do Not Resuscitate (DNR) Statements' include the following extract:

> It is appropriate to consider a DNR decision . . . where the patient's condition indicates that effective cardiopulmonary resuscitation is unlikely to be successful . . .

A report of the views of a group of oncology nurses[4] showed that they felt that resuscitation may be inappropriate if:

- it was unlikely to be successful
- resuscitation was not in agreement with the expressed wishes of a competent patient
- a valid advance directive refuses resuscitation
- successful resuscitation would result only in a poor quality of life.

This is a very difficult subject for you to discuss with the staff and your family. If such a discussion is suggested, it is because the staff need to be sure that everyone understands that they are aware of the feelings and agreed wishes of the whole family if such an unfortunate event should occur.

Think

☐	Why are you raising this topic now?
☐	Are you asking for euthanasia, or for treatment to be discontinued – 'allowing nature to take its course'?
☐	Are you really expressing a perceived lack of physical, emotional or spiritual support?
☐	Are you afraid of the process of dying?
☐	Is some outside pressure making you consider euthanasia?
☐	Do you feel that you are a burden on your family or carers?
☐	Are you depressed (*see* Chapter 11)?
☐	Do you feel a loss of dignity?

You also need to think about the doctors and nurses who are caring for you. Think about:

- their legal position
- their ethical position.

They will remind you of their legal position if the subject of euthanasia is raised. Breach of the law carries an automatic erasure from the General Medical Council register and the register of nurses, and the automatic loss of a job.

Ask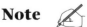

- If you are afraid of the process of dying, talk to the doctor or nurse about this. It is a common fear.
- If you are under pressure to ask about euthanasia, you can discuss this confidentially with the staff. They will be able to offer you appropriate advice and support. Hospices and palliative care units specialise in controlling symptoms and allowing patients to die with dignity in peaceful surroundings.
- If you feel that you are a burden on your family or carers, discuss this with your family and the nurse and doctor. Your family may need a break and a respite admission in the hospice may be a realistic option (*see* Chapter 41). Some relatives will not admit to needing to 'recharge their batteries' and need to be told that it is OK.
- Are you depressed? Talk to the doctor about this. You may need treatment.
- Do you feel a loss of dignity? Tell the doctor or nurse.
- Ask to speak to a minister or religious adviser if you feel that you are not ready to die and need to discuss religious and spiritual matters (*see* Chapter 43).

Note

If you have any specific requests about what should happen after your death, it might help for you to write these down and make sure that they are kept by a responsible person who can ensure they are carried out.

If you have any specific religious or cultural requirements regarding the handling of your body after death, that the staff may be unaware of, write these down clearly. Make sure that a senior member of staff is aware of your wishes.

Do

If you have specific requests about whether or not staff should try and resuscitate you, discuss these with a senior member of the staff. They will probably need a second person to be there as an independent witness.

Explore

The law and ethical views concerning euthanasia and the related issue of advance directives are very complex. You might wish to think about these situations:

- Is withdrawing, or not starting, a futile treatment euthanasia, or is it the most appropriate and ethical way to manage a patient's care?
- Are food and fluids delivered by a tube 'treatment'?

The law in many countries is changing and, as new cases come before the courts, our laws may change too.

More Information

A report in the British Medical Journal[5] showed that 80% of patients questioned wished to die with their symptoms relieved.

Another report, also in the British Medical Journal,[6] points out that good symptom control at the end of life might lead to fewer requests for euthanasia.

Palliative care is about trying to maximise quality of life without necessarily prolonging life. The staff will do their utmost to alleviate distressing symptoms – physical, social, emotional and spiritual.

References

1 Maughan T (2003) Euthanasia. *CMF Files number 23*. Christian Medical Fellowship, London.
2 Irwin M (2003) A new kind of living will. *Journal of the Royal Society of Medicine.* **96**: 411.
3 British Medical Association Resuscitation Council (UK) and Royal College of Nursing (2001) *Decisions Relating to Cardiopulmonary Resuscitation*. BMA.
4 Bass M (2003) Oncology nurses' perceptions of their role in resuscitation decisions. *Professional Nurse.* **18**(12): 710–13.
5 Clark J (2003) Freedom from unpleasant symptoms is essential for a good death. *BMJ.* **327**: 180.
6 Mak YYW, Elwyn G and Finlay IG (2003) Patients' voices are needed in debates on euthanasia. *BMJ.* **327**: 213–15.

Section 4

Appendices

Glossary of medical words used in the text

Acupressure
An ancient Chinese therapy involving pressure applied over various points on the body instead of the needles used in acupuncture.

Acupuncture
An ancient Chinese therapy involving the insertion of fine needles at various points on the body.

Advance directive
See living will.

Anaemia
Literally means 'bloodless'. The condition of having less red blood cells than normal owing to blood loss, lack of iron in the diet, or myelosuppression due to treatment for cancer.

Aromatherapy
A treatment involving the use of plant essential oils combined with gentle massage. The oils used by aromatherapists are highly concentrated and must only be used by trained staff. They are much more pure and concentrated than the cheap oils and burners sold in high street shops.

Bronchoscope
A rigid or flexible endoscope for inspecting the interior of the air passages to your lung, either for diagnostic purposes (e.g. biopsy) or for the removal of foreign bodies.

Bronchoscopy
Inspection of the interior of the air passages to your lungs through a bronchoscope.

Chemotherapy
The use of drugs to kill cancer cells. These are often given by injection or a drip into your veins, but may be given as tablets.

Denial
An unconscious defence mechanism used to allay anxiety by denying the existence of important conflicts or troublesome thoughts.

DNR
A short form of 'Do Not Resuscitate', a statement that might be written on the notes, indicating an agreement that the patient's condition indicates that effective cardiopulmonary resuscitation is unlikely to be successful.

Edema
See oedema.

Endoscope
A flexible instrument for the examination of the interior of a hollow part of the body, e.g. the bowel. The endoscope may carry a small camera and can also be used for taking small samples for further examination.

Endoscopy	Examination of the interior of a hollow part of the body, e.g. gullet or bowel, by means of an endoscope.
Euthanasia	The intentional putting to death of a person with an incurable or painful disease intended as an act of mercy.
Fistula	An abnormal passage from one surface to another surface – opening from both sides. (Compare sinus.)
Fungating	Growing exuberantly like a fungus or spongy growth.
Homoeopathy (sometimes spelled homeopathy)	A system of therapy, 'law of similia' (likes are cured by likes), which holds that a medicinal substance that can evoke certain symptoms in healthy individuals may be effective in the treatment of illnesses having symptoms closely resembling those produced by the substance.
Hydrotherapy	The use of water, often in a specially designed swimming pool, to assist with exercise and to strengthen weak muscles.
Jaundice	A yellowish staining of the eyes and skin, and associated with dark urine due to increased amounts of bile pigments in the blood.
Living will	Also called 'advance directives', these are the wishes of a person, recorded and witnessed at a time when they are in good health and of sound mind. The living will normally instructs that no attempt should be made to resuscitate the patient in the event of illness such that they are deprived of quality of life and become a burden on others for their care. Depending on its content, the document may have no legal status, or even request an act that is illegal in the UK.
Lymph	A clear, transparent, sometimes faintly yellow fluid that is collected from the tissues throughout the body, flows in the lymphatic vessels (through the lymph nodes), and is eventually added to the venous blood circulation.
Lymphoedema	Swelling (often of an arm or leg) as a result of obstruction of lymphatic vessels or lymph nodes and the accumulation of large amounts of lymph in the affected region.
Myelosuppression	A reduction in the normal function of your bone marrow. The bone marrow makes blood cells – red cells to carry oxygen, white cells to help fight infection. Myelosuppression is a side effect of many cancer treatments and results in reduced resistance to disease and can result in anaemia and subsequent shortness of breath.
Obturator	A specially designed denture used to close an opening of the roof of the mouth after surgery.

Oedema (edema in American texts)	An accumulation of an excessive amount of watery fluid in the tissues. This is usually seen as swollen ankles.
Pain assessment tools	These are a variety of numeric, verbal and visual scales designed to help you record the severity of your pain. To document the effect of any change in your medication, the assessment should be carried out on a regular basis until pain is controlled.
Palliative treatment	Treatment intended to relieve symptoms without curing the underlying disease.
Phantom limb	The sensation that an amputated limb is still present, often associated with painful abnormal sensations such as of burning, pricking, tickling, or tingling.
Radiotherapy	The use of high energy X-rays to kill cancer cells. Basically you lie very still on a table like an X-ray table. Treatment sessions usually last for a couple of minutes but may take several minutes to set up while you are positioned, etc.
Sinus	A cavity or hollow space. A sinus is a blind cul de sac that opens to one surface only. (Compare fistula.)
Tenesmus	An urgent desire to evacuate the bowel or bladder, involuntary straining, and the passage of little faecal matter or urine.
Tumour	The word tumour literally means any kind of abnormal lump, or growth, which may be benign (non-cancerous) or malignant (cancer) but in this book it refers specifically to a cancerous growth.

My personal pain record

This page can be copied and used to record and report your pain.

Date
When the pain started
What seemed to make it start/get worse
What relieved it
What it was like
How bad it was
How long it lasted
Where it was/where it went

Right   Left   Left   Right

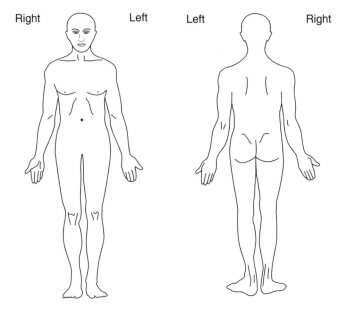

Fig. A2.1 Body diagrams for marking sites of pain.

Medication chart

You might wish to make up a chart like this to remind you of when to take your tablets. I have left lots of free spaces because things can change so often!

When to take my regular medications

Name of medication and what it's for	Times to be taken						
	6 a.m.	8 a.m.	10 a.m.	12 m.d.	2 p.m.	6 p.m.	10 p.m.

Medications to be taken if needed

Name of medication and what it's for	How often can I take it per 24 hours?	Tell the doctor or nurse if . . .

My notes

_____

_____

_____

Useful organisations

Acupuncturists	British Acupuncture Council
	Tel: 020 8735 0400
	Web site: www.acupuncture.org.uk
Aromatherapy	Aromatherapy Organisations Council
	PO Box 19834
	London SE25 6WF
	Tel: 020 8251 7912 (10 a.m.–2 p.m.)
	Provides a list of qualified practitioners in your area.
Bereavement	Cruse Bereavement Care
	Cruse House
	126 Sheen Road
	Richmond
	Surrey TW9 1UR
	Helpline: 0870 167 1677
	All types of bereavement counselling and a range of publications.
Bristol Cancer Help Centre	Grove House
	Cornwallis Grove
	Bristol BS8 4PG
	Information line: 0117 980 0500
	Provides a holistic approach to complementary care for cancer patients.
CancerBACUP	3 Bath Place
	Rivington Street
	London EC2A 3JR
	Tel: 020 7696 9003
	Web site: www.cancerbacup.org.uk
	Support and publications for patients, relatives and professionals.
Chiropractic	Chiropractic Patients' Association (CPA)
	Tel: 01722 415 027
	Web site: www.chiropractic.uk
	The General Chiropractic Council can help you find a chiropractor in your area.
	Tel: 0845 601 1796
	Web site: www.gcc.uk.org
Counselling	British Association for Counselling and Psychotherapy
	1 Regent Place
	Rugby
	Warwickshire CV21 2PJ
	Tel: 0870 443 5252
	Publishes a directory of counsellors in the UK.

DVLA	To check about notifiable medical conditions and see updated information from DVLA, look at their web site www.dvla.gov.uk/drivers/dmed1
Herbal practitioners	British Herbal Medicine Association Sun House Church Street Stroud Gloucestershire GL5 1JL Tel: 01453 751389 *Provides an information service and list of qualified herbal practitioners.*
Homoeopathy	The Faculty of Homoeopathy and British Homoeopathic Association Tel: 0870 444 3955 *Provides details of doctors and dentists who practise homoeopathy.*
Hospices	Hospice Information Service St Christopher's Hospice 51–59 Lawrie Park Road London SE26 6DZ Tel: 020 8778 9252 *Information about hospices and hospice care.*
Institute for Complementary Medicine	PO Box 194 London SE16 1QZ *Send an SAE with two loose stamps for information.*
Ireland – health advice	Web site: www.irishhealth.com *Free advice and information on-line and articles and resources on health in Ireland. All medical content is approved by Irish healthcare professionals.*
Lloyds Pharmacy	Home Health Hotline: 0845 607 4499 *Produce a 'Home Health Catalogue' which contains a selection of aids and appliances for people with disabilities and various health-related needs.*
Macmillan Cancerline	Tel: 0808 808 2020 (Monday–Friday 9 a.m.–5 p.m.) *Advice and information on all aspects of cancer.*
Macmillan Cancer Relief Information Line	Tel: 0845 601 6161
Marie Curie Cancer Care	89 Albert Embankment London SE1 7TP Tel: 020 7599 7777 (Scotland) 29A Albany Street Edinburgh EH1 3QN Tel: 0131 456 3700 *Home nursing service for day and night care.*

Questions to ask	The web site www.AskMe3.org suggests three simple questions patients should ask each time they see a health professional. They are: 'What is my main problem? What do I need to do? Why is it important to do this?'
Reflexologists	Association of Reflexologists 27 Old Gloucester Street London WC1N 3XX Tel: 0870 567 3320 *Provides a list of qualified practitioners in your area.*
St John Ambulance	Check telephone directory for local offices. *Advice about getting equipment on loan.*
Tak Tent Cancer Support Scotland	Tel: 0141 211 0122 *Information and support group network across Scotland.*
Tenovus Cancer Information Centre	Tel: 029 2019 6100 *A range of support services for people in Wales (available in English and Welsh).*